BRONCHIAL CARCINOMA

BRONCHIAL CARCINOMA

B. T. LE ROUX
CH.M., F.R.C.S.E.

Professor of Thoracic Surgery, University of Natal
Lately Senior Registrar and Clinical Tutor,
Thoracic Surgical Unit, Royal Infirmary, Edinburgh

Foreword by

A. LOGAN
M.A., F.R.C.S., F.R.C.S.E.

Senior Consultant Thoracic Surgeon, South East Region, Scotland
Reader in Thoracic Surgery, University of Edinburgh

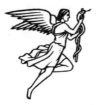

E. & S. LIVINGSTONE LTD
EDINBURGH AND LONDON
1968

©

E. & S. LIVINGSTONE LTD.
1968

SBN   443   00581   8

PRINTED IN GREAT BRITAIN

Foreword

IN the thirty-five years, almost a surgical lifetime, since Evarts Graham first resorted to pneumonectomy in its management, every feature of the natural history and surgical treatment of pulmonary carcinoma must have been recorded again and again. Reviews of very large numbers of cases have been made. The particular value of this series from Edinburgh is that besides being of considerable size it is homogeneous, derived from a fairly static population and managed by a few surgeons (the author among them) all trained in the same school and holding similar views. It has been recorded and analysed with precision and candour. For these reasons and also because it is a record of work from the unit with which I have been associated since its inception, to welcome Professor le Roux's monograph gives me pleasure.

ANDREW LOGAN

Edinburgh, 1968

Preface

AN accurate count was kept from the beginning of 1949 of the number of patients found by investigation in the Thoracic Surgical Unit in Edinburgh to have bronchial carcinoma. In July 1963 the number had reached 4,000, whereupon the case records which relate to these patients were scrutinised. Information for 193 patients was deficient to an extent which precluded inclusion in an analysis. A further 193 patients had been investigated by early December 1963, and these were therefore included in the series, which now extended over very nearly 15 years. The purpose of this monograph is to review presentation, natural history, management and the results of management of 4,000[1] of 4,193 consecutive cases of bronchial carcinoma. Omission from the analysis of the 193 incompletely documented records is thought likely not significantly to bias conclusions drawn from an assessment of results of management; but so far as can be ascertained, none of the 193 patients was managed surgically, so that the proportion of patients suitable for surgical management in this series is fractionally too high—61 of the last-included 193 patients were managed surgically. Since the difference in a series of this magnitude is only 0·3 per cent, this too is unlikely significantly to modify conclusions. The patients whose case records were reviewed represent all patients seen with bronchial carcinoma, whether or not they were managed surgically. Follow-up in those managed surgically is complete, and in those unsuitable for surgical management, very nearly complete.

While this review includes all but 193 patients seen in a Unit over most of 15 years, it is not presented as a review of bronchial carcinoma in the region served by this unit in the period under review. In the latter half of the period a small but increasing number of patients with bronchial carcinoma were managed surgically in a second unit in the region; for nearly 10 of the 15 years detailed investigation of patients with respiratory disease was undertaken by a medical unit in the region, and those patients with bronchial carcinoma found unsuitable for surgical management were not necessarily seen in a surgical unit; and all patients with bronchial carcinoma in the region were not inevitably seen in any of these units, or recognised as having bronchial carcinoma before death in other wards, or in other hospitals in the region. The 4,000 patients reviewed probably represent between half and two-thirds of the number of cases of bronchial carcinoma amongst the population of $1\frac{1}{2}$ million in the South East Region of Scotland during the period under review. There may be a surgical bias to this series, but in the earlier years the number of patients managed surgically in relation to the total number seen was proportionately similar to that in later years, and the number of patients seen each year has not greatly changed. Moreover, in this group of 4,000 patients, most of the reported and widely varied aspects

[1] Mr. Gordon Jack reviewed 668 cases seen between May 1946 and December 1951, and some of these cases are, therefore, included in the present series (Jack, G. D. (1952-53) Bronchogenic carcinoma). *Trans. med-chir. Soc. Edinb.*, Session CXXXII, p. 75.

of the disease have been encountered, so that it is probable that the review supplies a reasonably complete assessment of the natural and therapeutically modified history of the disease.

The short, pithy title required of modern books has taken the place of the discursive title which gave the prospective reader some insight into the contents, and limitations, of the volume. But it is regrettably necessary to conform, if only for reasons of economy. The appropriate extended title for this monograph would be "An Analysis of Presentation and Clinical Behaviour in 4,000 Cases of Bronchial Carcinoma with Observations regarding the Influence of Age, Histological Type, and Surgical Management in Selected Cases, on Prognosis".

The monograph is not illustrated with radiographic reproductions. In recent years (1964 and 1968) two Portfolios of Chest Radiographs have been published[1] in which are illustrated all the common and many of the unusual radiographic manifestations of bronchial carcinoma, and it seems unnecessary to transpose from these readily available publications radiographs which would serve to increase the bulk and cost of this monograph.

The material presented is factual, and, where necessary, reference has been made to other works which serve to support or augment conclusions. But on the whole, the material is presented simply as factual, and as a source of reference for others who may wish to lend weight to their own conclusions. A criticism which could be levelled at this monograph is the paucity of reference to other works. The literature which relates to bronchial carcinoma has reached proportions which can justifiably be called astronomical. To incorporate relevant references to so vast a reservoir of facts, most well-documented elsewhere, is an undertaking of some magnitude. The analysis of the series of cases on which this monograph is based has itself proved a considerable task, and its publication fully three years after completion of a personal scrutiny of case records, a survey of surviving patients, and a search through registers of deaths, and other sources of information reflects the time that it has taken to present the facts, let alone compare the figures with other series. The monograph must, therefore, serve as an analysis of a group of patients in a conveniently portable form to which those whose penchant it is to compare and contrast may have recourse.

To detail the results of surgical management is inescapable but tedious. Of more interest to physicians will, it is thought, be the effects on prognosis of such factors as age; histology; presentation without symptoms and with an abnormality found at routine radiography; presentation because of hypertrophic pulmonary osteoarthropathy; the influence of pleural effusion on the results of management; the incidence of unnecessary pulmonary resection or pulmonary resection of unnecessary magnitude, in the belief that a pulmonary lesion is a carcinoma; the pattern of emergence of metastases, and similar information not wholly surgical. The first chapter is intended as a precis in

[1] *A Portfolio of Chest Radiographs* and *A Second Portfolio of Chest Radiographs*. E. & S. Livingstone, Edinburgh.

which the natural and surgically modified history of bronchial carcinoma as encountered in 4,000 cases is outlined. This chapter is transposed with little change from *A Second Portfolio of Chest Radiographs*. Subsequent chapters are intended to stand alone, and each represents an individual article already published or suitable for separate publication. There is, therefore, inevitable repetition—it is, for example, necessary to record that hypertrophic pulmonary osteoarthropathy is associated with adenocarcinoma disproportionately often both in the section devoted to bronchial carcinoma with hypertrophic pulmonary osteoarthropathy and that devoted to histology, and to relate mortality in the post-operative period to age both in the chapter devoted to the influence of age on prognosis, and that in which surgical management is discussed.

The case records on which this monograph is based are held in the archives of the Thoracic Surgical Unit in the Royal Infirmary in Edinburgh. While the author has had a hand in the management of nearly all the patients to whom these records relate, they were all referred to Mr. Andrew Logan, and in their surgical management he, Mr. David Wade, Mr. R. J. McCormack, Mr. Philip Walbaum and a number of surgical registrars in training, were intimately concerned. This monograph is a record of the management of bronchial carcinoma in a particular Unit by an almost unchanging team, whose attitude towards and whose management of the disease has remained remarkably consistent. It is a record of the work of a unit, and not in any way an individual effort. Where there is the need to draw conclusions and make pronouncements, the views expressed are those held by the unit, and again are not individual.

Permission for reproduction in this monograph of some of the material which appears in the following papers has been given by the Editors of the Journals concerned, and this permission is gratefully acknowledged: *Thorax* (" Bronchial Carcinoma "); *Journal of the Royal Colleges of Surgeons of Edinburgh* (" Management of Bronchial Carcinoma by Segmental Resection " and " The Incidence of Pulmonary Resection undertaken with a Provisional and later Unsubstantiated Diagnosis of Bronchial Carcinoma "); *Geriatrics* (" The Influence of Age on the Results of Management of Bronchial Carcinoma "); *Scottish Medical Journal* (" The Presentation of Bronchial Carcinoma " and " The Influence of Predominant Cell Type on the Management and Prognosis of Bronchial Carcinoma "); *South African Medical Journal* (" Bronchial Carcinoma with Pleural Effusion " and " Bronchial Carcinoma with Hypertrophic Pulmonary Osteoarthropathy ").

Part of the expense incurred in making this survey was defrayed by a grant from the South East Regional Hospital Board, Scotland, and the Royal Infirmary, Edinburgh. I am grateful to them, and to Messrs. E. & S. Livingstone for undertaking publication, particularly since there is available, from the same house of publishers, a monograph[1] in which similar material from many sources is similarly dealt with.

[1] *Carcinoma of the Lung.* Edited by J. R. Bignall. E. & S. Livingstone, Edinburgh, 1958.

Contents

CONTENTS

I

General

FROM a retrospective analysis of the case records of 4,000 patients managed over a period of 15 years and established sooner or later to have bronchial carcinoma, it is possible to make certain generalisations.[1]

Bronchial carcinoma is more common in men—only 10 per cent of patients are women. The highest incidence of the disease is in the sixth and seventh decades; 10 per cent of patients are 70 years or older when first they are seen; about one fifth of women and fewer than one sixth of men with bronchial carcinoma are younger than 50 years at the time of first investigation. While the yearly incidence of the disease does not appear to be changing significantly the incidence amongst those over 70 years is rising and amongst those under 50 years may be falling. An increasing incidence of the disease in the aged is probably explicable on the grounds of a generally aging population: a diminishing incidence in the younger age group is recorded in other series, and an explanation for the fact is lacking.

The survey, of which this is a summary, was made in a region where coal mining is a common occupation and of the patients in this series 15 per cent were coal miners, an occupational incidence which is disproportionately high. It is generally maintained that coal mining does not predispose specifically to bronchial carcinoma. That a large number of coalminers were found to have bronchial carcinoma may be related to the fact that theirs is an occupational group regularly examined radiographically and probably more often than are most other occupational groups.

Of every four patients with bronchial carcinoma three are known to have been cigarette smokers and most of these were heavy smokers. Of the total number of patients 3 per cent smoked only a pipe and 4 per cent claimed never to have smoked: amongst the women in the series 15 per cent claimed never to have smoked. Latterly there has emerged a noticeable reluctance among patients to admit that they smoke. In one third of those who did not smoke the tumour was squamous. The smoking habits of 20 per cent of patients is not known, an incidence of omission in the records probably significant of the percentage of failure adequately to record in all other aspects of the anamnesis, and perhaps an argument in favour of demanding, from rotational junior staff who interrogate patients, the completion of a detailed

[1] Le Roux, B. T. (1968). Bronchial carcinoma. *Thorax,* **23,** 136.

1

pro forma rather than the recording of answers to those variable questions which they may remember to ask. While it has been clearly established that a large proportion of those patients who develop bronchial carcinoma have smoked cigarettes for some years, the precise relationship between cigarette smoking and bronchial carcinoma is not yet established. It is also clear that not smoking is not a guarantee against the development even of squamous carcinoma, and that cigarette smoking is not the only cause of bronchial carcinoma.

Patients shown by investigation to have bronchial carcinoma presented in one of five ways: (1) With one, some or all of the cardinal symptoms of respiratory disease—cough, sputum, haemoptysis, chest pain, dyspnoea and wheeze. (2) Without symptoms and because of an abnormality detected on a chest radiograph made for routine purposes—during mass miniature radiographic surveys; during radiographic surveys among coal-miners and other occupational groups; during the routine follow-up of patients known to have had pulmonary tuberculosis; for insurance or immigration purposes; and so on. (3) Because of evidence of extension of or metastases from bronchial carcinoma, e.g. cerebral or osseous metastases; hoarseness of voice; obstruction of the superior vena cava; jaundice. (4) With non-specific symptoms such as loss of weight and appetite, insomnia, dyspepsia and so on. (5) With what may be called the humoral or neural concomitants of the disease—hypertrophic pulmonary osteoarthropathy; myopathy and neuropathy; and possibly others such as Cushing's syndrome.

Cough was a symptom in three of every four patients with bronchial carcinoma and in 40 per cent cough was severe and one of the primary reasons for medical advice being sought. Cough was, in nearly all instances, at some time productive. In many patients cough was not a new symptom and was often attributed to smoking. Worsening of an otherwise chronic cough, often in relation to one or several febrile episodes, was a common history.

Haemoptysis was a symptom in more than half (57 per cent), and in 4 per cent of patients haemoptysis was the only symptom. Presentation for investigation in 1 per cent was prompted by a single haemoptysis. In patients with haemoptysis this symptom varied from occasional to daily. The complaint of daily haemoptysis—usually in the form of blood-streaking of the sputum in the early morning—was regarded as typical of bronchial carcinoma. There was commonly delay, even amongst doctors later shown to have bronchial carcinoma, of months rather than weeks before patients with the complaint of haemoptysis presented for investigation. Delay in investigation of haemoptysis by a thoracic surgeon was commonly occasioned both by delay in referral for a surgical opinion, and delay on the part of the patient to report the abnormality.

Pain related to bronchial carcinoma was not usually acute pleural pain and was commonly an intermittent ache, which lasted for hours at a time, was worse at night and aggravated by posture, and relieved by activity. Severe pain was common in those patients shown by investigation to have invasion of

2

the chest wall, but chest wall invasion, vertebral invasion, and rib and vertebral metastases were found in patients who denied pain, and the complaint of pain was not uncommon in patients found to have pulmonary tumours which were successfully managed surgically and in whom pain could not be related to pleural invasion or infection.

It was often not possible to equate the complaint of dyspnoea with diminution in measured respiratory function; very nearly normal respiratory function figures were recorded in patients amongst whose more distressing complaints was dyspnoea; there was little relationship between the size of a radiographic opacity (and presumably, therefore, the extent of deprivation of functioning lung), and the severity of the dyspnoea.

One in every four patients with bronchial carcinoma gave a history either of an acute febrile respiratory illness, often called influenza, from which recovery had been slow and incomplete, or of a series of acute febrile illnesses with complete or incomplete recovery between episodes. Cough with purulent sputum, chest pain, dyspnoea and haemoptysis were often features of these acute illnesses, but evanescent features of which little cognisance had been taken during the acute episode—in fact these features were taken for granted as part of the acute episode. This history—of failure to make an anticipated recovery from an acute respiratory illness—is accepted as strongly suggestive of the diagnosis of bronchial carcinoma in the same way as is daily haemoptysis.

Wheeze was a presenting symptom in 2 per cent of patients and in those who were not chronic asthmatics the complaint of wheeze could usually be related to a tumour which had extended in a main bronchus close to the main carina, and even into the trachea; and as a prognostic feature, wheeze, like stridor, was often significant of inoperability. Stridor, as distinct from wheeze was less common and fewer than 1 per cent of patients were admitted to hospital urgently stridulous and in need of therapeutic bronchoscopy, at which tumour had to be cored from the trachea or both main bronchi in order to establish a more adequate airway. While stridor with bronchial carcinoma is often a herald of death, it is important to remember that acute tracheo-bronchitis even in an adult may present with stridor as evidence of gross proximal airway obstruction, and always to investigate stridor by bronchoscopy.

There was a group of patients—some 15 per cent of the total number—who presented not with respiratory symptoms but with symptoms such as loss of weight and appetite; tiredness and lassitude; non-specific general ill health; dyspepsia; with recent difficulty in the control of previously easily managed diabetes, and so on. In these patients referral to a thoracic surgical unit was usually the result of an abnormality having been detected on a chest radiograph made as one of many routine investigations undertaken in a search for a cause for non-specific symptoms, or because an abnormality had been recognised during routine fluoroscopy of the chest as part of a barium study.

Nearly 2 per cent of patients with bronchial carcinoma had at the time of their first presentation the complaint of dysphagia and in half of these dysphagia was the presenting complaint. Whatever the breakdown may be of

3

the causes of dysphagia amongst the population at large, of those patients referred to a thoracic surgical unit a common cause of dysphagia is a malignant tumour in the proximal part of the alimentary tract. Dysphagia from malignant disease, moreover, is very nearly always the consequence of a primary alimentary tumour. Where dysphagia is the consequence of metastatic malignant disease, the primary tumour is very nearly always bronchial, and the only other common source of mediastinal glandular metastases which compress the oesophagus is mammary carcinoma.

A small group of patients presented with the complaint of recurrent peripheral venous thromboses, often called thrombophlebitis migrans. In this group of patients the incidence of operability was lower than average, the incidence of metastases at operation higher than average, the incidence of death from pulmonary embolism in convalescence from an operation remarkably high, and that of long survival remarkably low.

Bronchial carcinoma was found in patients in whom presentation was with a myopathy or neuropathy; because of Cushing's syndrome; because of exfoliative dermatitis, dermatomyositis or purpura; and with other evidence of general systemic disease. A great deal of research, much of it successful, has been devoted to establishing a connection between bronchial carcinoma and presentation in these unusual ways. It is important to remember to search for bronchial carcinoma in a patient who presents with spontaneous pneumothorax. The patient who presents to a general surgical charge with an inguinal hernia and who has a chronic cough may well have a bronchial carcinoma. Cough syncope and cough fractures may be the form of presentation in men with bronchial carcinoma.

Apart from a small number of patients, too ill at the time of admission to hospital to withstand routine investigations, or who died before investigations could be completed, all patients were submitted to a routine series of investigations. History and clinical examinations were recorded. Routine chest radiographs were made and all patients well enough to go to the X-ray department were examined fluoroscopically, primarily to search for evidence of phrenic paresis and displacement of the barium-filled oesophagus. Tomograms and other special films were made in circumstances in which they were believed necessary, for diagnostic or record purposes. Bronchoscopy was a routine and it was the practice to make a biopsy from a visible tumour. In 58 per cent of patients the diagnosis of bronchial carcinoma was established at bronchoscopy. The tumours in these patients were called " central "—on the ground of visibility at bronchoscopy. In the remaining patients the appearances at bronchoscopy were normal or bronchi were displaced but with the mucosa normal, and these patients were recorded as having tumours of " peripheral " type. The purpose of bronchography is to demonstrate dilated bronchi and bronchography was not regarded as contributory in establishing the diagnosis of bronchial carcinoma. There are too many other causes, of which mucus is the commonest, of obstruction of bronchi beyond the range of bronchoscopic vision to justify acceptance of bronchographic evidence of peripheral bronchial obstruction as evidence of carcinoma. Pleural effusion in relation to bronchial carcinoma was investigated by thoracentesis, examination of the pleural liquid both bacteriologically and histologically, the replacement of the effusion with air, thoracoscopy and pleural biopsy under vision. Biopsies were made of palpable cervical lymph nodes and from other easily accessible metastases—in skin, subcutaneous and other soft tissues and in muscle. Sputum was routinely examined for tumour cells, but often not by an expert specifically trained in the techniques involved. Symptoms such as bone pain, haematuria, and so on, were appropriately investigated; a search was not routinely made in symptomless patients for cryptic metastases, by radiographic skeletal surveys, by routine pyelography, or similar techniques. Special examinations, such as pneumomediastinography, were occasionally undertaken in unusual circumstances, but were never a part of routine investigation. Respiratory function—in particular the forced expiratory volume—was measured in patients in whom surgical management was contemplated, but was rarely found more informative than crude assessment of exercise tolerance, say by climbing stairs. An electrocardiogram was made pre-operatively in all patients over the age of 40 years. Routine pre-operative chest radiographs—made on the day before operation—were usually anteroposterior films made with portable radiographic apparatus with the patient in bed, to provide a more precise base line against which to judge post-operative films. A search for tubercle bacilli was made in serial specimens of sputum from all patients.

With regard to the radiographic appearances of bronchial carcinoma, in only three of 4,000 patients were postero-anterior and lateral radiographs normal—repeatedly normal, and normal to a number of independent experts. Presentation in these three patients was with haemoptysis, in one associated with wheeze. The tumours were visible at bronchoscopy, in a main bronchus in all, and also in the trachea in one. Tubercle bacilli were found in the sputum of nearly 2 per cent of patients with pulmonary carcinoma and cavitated pulmonary tuberculosis was recognised radiographically as a concomitant of bronchial carcinoma in 1 per cent of patients, bilaterally and as a bar to surgical management of carcinoma, in some of these. The radiographic changes of pneumoconiosis were commonplace and the radiographic features of progressive massive fibrosis were recognised in 1 per cent of patients. Pleural effusion was a concomitant of bronchial carcinoma in 10 per cent. Obstructive emphysema, the consequence of bronchial carcinoma, was surprisingly uncommon.

In 7 per cent of patients with bronchial carcinoma there were related cardiovascular abnormalities, sufficiently gross in one tenth of these to preclude surgical management. Operative mortality was quadrupled in those with systemic hypertension with electrocardiographic changes, or with a history of angina on effort, or in those who had previously had a myocardial infarct. Of those patients in whom cardiovascular disease and bronchial carcinoma coexisted, who were managed surgically and who died in convalescence, half died from an acute cardiovascular episode—myocardial infarction, or in acute congestive cardiac failure.

Of all patients with bronchial carcinoma, 55 per cent were unsuitable for surgical management when first they were seen, most because of clinical, radiographic, fluoroscopic or bronchoscopic evidence of metastases and the remainder because of evidence other than metastases of unsuitability for surgical management, or because of death during investigation. The remaining patients—45 per cent—were regarded, after investigation, as suitable for management by exploratory thoracotomy with a view to resection of pulmonary carcinoma. Nearly one fifth of these patients—8 per cent of the total—were found to have a tumour the resection of which was technically impossible or therapeutically pointless; and pulmonary resection was completed in approximately 37 per cent of the total. Pneumonectomy was undertaken twice as often as lobectomy.

The pulmonary tumour in about 55 per cent of patients with bronchial carcinoma was squamous in type. Undifferentiated tumours including " oat cell " carcinoma accounted for approximately 40 per cent of the series. Adenocarcinoma is relatively uncommon and in most series accounts for less than 10 per cent and in this series for no more than 5 per cent of the total. Alveolar cell or bronchiolar carcinoma is rare, and accounted for less than 1 per cent. In any large series mixed tumours are common—that is, tumours in which a biopsy from the primary may be called squamous, sections of the whole tumour may show different histological varieties, mediastinal or cervical glandular metastases may be undifferentiated, and a hepatic or cerebral metastasis found at necropsy may show the histological morphology of, say, adenocarcinoma. All possible permutations of the histological varieties may be found in the same primary tumour and in metastases. Oat cell carcinoma is said to be the tumour, the histological appearance of which is most consistent throughout the primary and in metastases.

Amongst those tumours found suitable for management by pulmonary resection, most were squamous; amongst those tumours found unsuitable for management by exploratory thoracotomy, the number of undifferentiated tumours was in excess of the number of squamous tumours. The operative mortality of exploratory thoracotomy without pulmonary resection was 6 per cent. Nearly three quarters of patients found by exploration to have an irresectable pulmonary carcinoma had died within a year of operation. Nearly half the patients, in whom management of pulmonary carcinoma was by pneumonectomy, were found to have hilar glandular metastases. The operative mortality of pneumonectomy was 12 per cent, and the operative mortality rate increased significantly with age, being 20 per cent in those 65 years or older. For reasons unconvincingly explained the operative mortality for right pneumonectomy was nearly twice that of left pneumonectomy. The three common causes of death in the post-operative period after pneumonectomy were pulmonary infection, coronary thrombosis and pulmonary embolism—together accounting for three quarters of the deaths in this group. Survival rate in the first three years after pneumonectomy for pulmonary carcinoma was significantly higher in those for whom resection was undertaken for squamous carcinoma than in those for whom resection was undertaken for undifferentiated carcinoma. Thereafter survival rates for the two types of tumour ran a roughly parallel course. One in every three patients who died from metastases in the first two years after pneumonectomy died with cerebral metastases. Of all patients in whom bronchial carcinoma was managed by pneumonectomy 20 per cent were alive more than five years after operation. While most of those who survived a long time were not shown to have mediastinal glandular metastases at operation, the finding of metastases in mediastinal glands is not a bar to long survival. Following pulmonary resection for bronchial carcinoma, survival for more than five years is not an insurance against the development of metastases at a later date, or the growth of a new primary tumour.

In nearly 70 per cent of those patients in whom bronchial carcinoma was managed by lobectomy, the tumour was squamous in type. The overall operative mortality for lobectomy was approximately half that of pneumonectomy and was 14 per cent in those 65 years and older, and more than 20 per cent in those 70 years and older. For unexplained reasons right upper lobectomy was the operation with the highest mortality rate; " sleeve " resection—usually of the right upper lobe with part of the stem bronchus—was a variety of lobectomy free from complications. The long survival rate after lobectomy for bronchial carcinoma was twice that for pneumonectomy. The fact that lobectomy for carcinoma is less commonly complicated by death in early convalescence and more commonly followed by long survival than is pneumonectomy does not establish lobectomy for carcinoma as a " better " operation than pneumonectomy. When a pulmonary carcinoma is manageable by lobectomy the prognosis is better, mainly because of the small size of the tumour, which in turn relates to the biology of the tumour and the rate of growth, or early and therefore often chance recognition, and to the position of the tumour in relation to the pulmonary hilum.

Bronchial carcinoma in a very small number of patients was managed by segmental resection. Segmental resection is not generally regarded as an acceptable alternative to, say, lobectomy in the management of established bronchial carcinoma, and the circumstances in which segmental resection was undertaken were unusual. Pulmonary carcinoma managed by segmental resection is always peripheral in type and the lesion is often interpreted, by palpation at thoracotomy, as tuberculous, on the grounds of hardness, related scarring or multiplicity of nodules. Occasionally the segment in which the tumour lies is separated from neighbouring segments by an anatomically complete fissure—usually the apical segment of a lower lobe or the lingular segment of the left upper lobe—and in these circumstances it may be judged as effective to manage the tumour by segmental resection as by lobectomy. In even rarer circumstances severe limitation of respiratory reserve in patients in whom thoracotomy is undertaken with a view to making the most limited resection possible to establish the diagnosis of carcinoma, may be an indication for management of a peripheral pulmonary lesion by segmental resection. It is factual that, amongst patients in whom bronchial carcinoma was managed by segmental resection— and in all these patients the tumour was small and peripheral—long survival was relatively as common as that after pneumonectomy, and late death was more commonly the consequence of coronary artery insufficiency or respiratory failure than of metastases.

Those patients who presented without symptoms, and with an abnormality detected on a chest radiograph made for an unrelated purpose, were more often suitable for surgical management of bronchial carcinoma than were those who presented because of symptoms—but not all were suitable for surgical management. In this group of patients the number with peripheral tumours was substantially higher and the number with undifferentiated tumours substantially lower than amongst those who presented with symptoms. Approximately one quarter of those who presented without symptoms and with an abnormality demonstrated on a routine chest radiograph made for unrelated purpose were unsuitable for or declined surgical management. Operative mortality and the rate of irresectability at exploratory thoracotomy—both about 5 per cent— were lower than amongst those in whom bronchial carcinoma had unequivocally declared itself before radiological investigations were undertaken.

It was stated earlier that some 45 per cent of patients, when first they presented for investigation, were found to have clinical, radiographic, fluoroscopic, bronchoscopic or thoracoscopic evidence of metastases or extrapulmonary extension of pulmonary carcinoma, which made them unsuitable for surgical management. Cervical lymph glandular metastasis was the commonest single clinical evidence of dissemination of bronchial carcinoma. In approximately 10 per cent of all patients with pulmonary carcinoma, cervical nodes only on the same side as the primary tumour were the site of metastases. In approximately 2 per cent cervical glandular metastases were bilateral and in another 2 per cent cervical glandular metastases were only contra-lateral. In nearly half those with ipsilateral cervical glandular metastasis this was the only evidence of metastases on standard clinical and special investigation. Where cervical glands were palpable in patients with bronchial carcinoma, these were found by biopsy to be the site of metastasis in three of every four patients. Scalene node biopsy in patients in whom a gland could not be felt was established as an unrewarding exercise. Cervical glandular metastasis from a left pulmonary primary, not only in the lower lobe, to the right side of the neck was not importantly more common than was a metastasis from a right pulmonary primary carcinoma to the left side of the neck. Bilateral cervical glandular metastases were only occasionally the only evidence of spread of bronchial carcinoma, and most patients with bilateral cervical glandular metastases died within a few weeks of investigation.

Axillary lymph glandular metastasis from bronchial carcinoma without chest wall invasion was very rarely the only clinical evidence of metastasis and, in two patients, the primary tumour and the invaded axillary glands were on opposite sides. A radiographic opacity in the vicinity of the azygos vein and

8

inseparable from the mediastinum, in patients in whom the pulmonary primary is right or left sided, is good evidence of lymph glandular metastasis and of unsuitability for surgical management. Where the radiographic appearances were those of lymphangitis carcinomatosa, dyspnoea was usually the predominant symptom and death was usually rapid. Unilateral radiographic features of lymphangitis carcinomatosa were more commonly right-sided than left; where the changes were bilateral there was usually a right-sided predominance; unilateral radiographic features of lymphangitis carcinomatosa are almost always evidence of spread from a primary pulmonary tumour rather than from an extra-thoracic primary tumour.

Some 3 per cent of patients found on detailed investigation to have pulmonary carcinoma presented because of cerebral metastases. Hemiplegia, epilepsy and personality changes were the three most common forms of presentation; speech defects, cerebellar symptoms and headache were other common presenting symptoms. Only once was it found rewarding to excise a cerebral metastasis and thereafter to manage surgically the pulmonary primary. Where suspicion, however slight, is raised regarding the existence of cerebral metastasis, the presence of which is unconfirmed by detailed investigation, the passage of time, often brief, usually confirms the suspicion.

Approximately 2 per cent of patients were found to have osseous metastases as the only evidence of dissemination of bronchial carcinoma at the time of their first investigation; three in every four of these patients presented with the complaint of bone pain and without new respiratory symptoms. The commonest sites of osseous metastases were the ribs and the vertebrae. In approximately the same percentage of patients hepatic metastases were found as the only evidence of spread of tumour at the time of first investigation.

Nearly 5 per cent of patients presented with the clinical features of obstruction of the superior vena cava. More of these patients were women, of a younger than average age, and the incidence of undifferentiated tumours was higher, than amongst those who presented in other ways. Obstruction of the superior vena cava and cervical lymph glandular metastases, bilateral disproportionately often, were commonly associated. A right vocal cord palsy in patients with bronchial carcinoma is rare, and when it is found it is usually in association with obstruction of the superior vena cava, a right upper pulmonary carcinoma and right cervical lymph glandular metastases. It was usually possible quickly to relieve the symptoms and signs of obstruction of the superior vena cava by irradiation; the recurrence of caval obstruction was common and usually a herald of death. Obstruction of the superior vena cava was nearly always associated with a right-sided pulmonary carcinoma, usually in the right upper lobe.

Fluoroscopy demonstrated, in approximately 5 per cent of patients, that bronchial carcinoma was unsuitable for surgical management—more often because of displacement of the barium-filled oesophagus than because of interruption of a phrenic nerve. Interruption of the left recurrent laryngeal nerve as evidence of mediastinal invasion was found in approximately 4 per cent of patients. The pulmonary opacity in patients with a left recurrent laryngeal nerve palsy was left-sided in nearly all and in the left upper lobe or at the left pulmonary hilum in most. Histological confirmation of the diagnosis of bronchial carcinoma was achieved, at the time of their first investigation, in only about a third of patients who presented with a left cord palsy. Where the histology of the tumour was sooner or later established, squamous tumours predominated. Survival time from the onset of hoarseness of voice was often surprisingly long. Irradiation of a pulmonary carcinoma in patients with hoarseness of voice will not restore the voice.

Proximal extension of tumour, seen at bronchoscopy and usually established by biopsy, precluded surgical management of pulmonary carcinoma in nearly 5 per cent of patients. Bronchial carcinoma is judged unsuitable for surgical management where the main carina is seen to be invaded or where the main carina, while not ulcerated, is unequivocally broad and the main bronchi are splayed; where the trachea is involved, unless this involvement is limited to the right lateral wall, and this is usually found in relation to a tumour of the right upper bronchus; where the trachea is compressed or scabbard-shaped; where the tumour can be demonstrated histologically to involve bronchi, usually the main bronchi, of both sides; where tumour obstructs a main bronchus, within $\frac{1}{2}$ cm. of the main carina on the right and within $1\frac{1}{2}$ cm. of the main carina on the left, provided that involvement of this degree of proximity is unequivocally medial and not only lateral; and where, by the independent assessment of two experts, a main bronchus is found to be abnormally rigid—an assessment rarely accepted as the only basis for not undertaking surgical management in a patient suitable in all other respects for this form of treatment. Adenocarcinoma rarely extended proximally in the ways outlined. A disproportionately large number of tumours which extended proximally were right-sided.

Invasion of the chest wall, not uncommonly unsuspected clinically, was recognised radiographically in some 3 per cent of patients. In a third of these resection was undertaken because chest wall invasion was lateral; in another third the tumour was apical and associated with the features of Pancoast's syndrome; in the last third invasion was medial, either anteriorly or posteriorly.

Where pleural effusion is associated with pulmonary carcinoma, this is routinely investigated by thoracoscopy. This technique demonstrated the presence of pleural metastases as the only evidence of extra-pulmonary extension of bronchial carcinoma in approximately 2 per cent of patients. Half the patients with pleural metastases had peripheral tumours, and a disproportionately large number were women. Adenocarcinoma metastasised to the pleura disproportionately often. Most patients with pleural metastases died within six months of the diagnosis having been made, in contra-distinction to patients with primary pleural tumours in whom long survival is not uncommon. Pleural effusion, even if sanguinous, in association with bronchial carcinoma, is not synonymous with pleural metastases and is an indication for investigation, not a reason for despair.

10

Hypertrophic pulmonary osteoarthropathy was a concomitant of bronchial carcinoma in approximately 1 per cent of patients. In this group of patients the tumour was found disproportionately often to be an adenocarcinoma. The incidence of peripheral tumours and the rate of resectability amongst patients who presented with hypertrophic pulmonary osteoarthropathy was disproportionately high, and the incidence of long survival disproportionately low. Resection of the pulmonary lesion, or irradiation, relieved joint pain. The appearance of intra-thoracic recurrence or metastases in the late post-operative period was, in a small proportion of the patients who presented originally with hypertrophic pulmonary osteoarthropathy, associated with a return of the symptoms and signs of this concomitant of bronchial carcinoma, but this phenomenon was never observed in patients who had not initially presented with hypertrophic osteoarthropathy and who later developed intra-thoracic metastases.

Diminished respiratory reserve constituted the only bar to the surgical management of bronchial carcinoma in approximately 3 per cent of patients. More than three quarters of the patients in this group were older than 59 years when first they were seen, whereas in the series as a whole, fewer than half the patients were older than 59 years. In elderly patients with poor respiratory reserve and small peripheral tumours, death, more often than not, was with rather than from bronchial carcinoma. In approximately another 4 per cent of patients there was found a non-metastatic contra-indication to surgical management other than diminution in respiratory reserve—for example, extensive pulmonary tuberculosis, chronic asthma, gross pneumoconiosis, bullous emphysema, myocardial disease, advanced age alone, or frailty.

Approximately 2 per cent of patients who were being investigated for a lesion later established to be a bronchial carcinoma, died before investigations could be completed. In many of these patients the terminal event was not directly attributable to bronchial carcinoma; most at necropsy had evidence of widespread metastases. Techniques used in the investigation of 4,000 patients with bronchial carcinoma resulted in the death of two patients—a mortality from investigation of 0·05 per cent.

II

Presentation

SUMMARY

Bronchial carcinoma in 4,000 patients investigated over a 15 year period, presented in these ways[1]:

1. With some or all of the cardinal symptoms of respiratory disease (68 per cent). Daily haemoptysis and recurrent febrile respiratory illnesses with complete or incomplete recovery between episodes, were two manners of presentation particularly suggestive of the diagnosis of bronchial carcinoma.

2. Without symptoms and because of an abnormality detected on a chest radiograph made for routine purposes (5 per cent).

3. With evidence of extension of or metastases from bronchial carcinoma without respiratory symptoms or with respiratory symptoms long accepted and not recently changed (13 per cent). Evidence of extension of bronchial carcinoma was established by investigation in 45 per cent of the whole series.

4. With non-specific symptoms such as loss of weight, dyspepsia and so on, and without respiratory symptoms (12 per cent).

5. With unusual symptoms which were not respiratory, or with humoral or neural concomitants of bronchial carcinoma such as hypertrophic pulmonary osteoarthropathy without, or with only unobtrusive, respiratory symptoms (2 per cent).

The incidence of bronchial carcinoma amongst coal miners in the South East Region of Scotland may be disproportionately high.

THE patients in this series presented in a number of ways which can be grouped thus: (1) With one, some or all of the cardinal symptoms of respiratory disease—cough, sputum, haemoptysis, chest pain, dyspnoea and wheeze. (2) Without symptoms, and because of an abnormality detected on a chest radiograph made for routine purposes—during mass miniature radiographic surveys; during radiographic surveys amongst coal miners; during the routine follow-up of patients known to have had pulmonary tuberculosis; for insurance or immigration purposes; and many others. If there is a significantly higher incidence of bronchial carcinoma amongst coal miners, this may be related to the fact that this occupational group is examined routinely radiographically probably more often than most other occupational groups. (3) Primarily because of evidence of extension of or metastases from bronchial carcinoma—cerebral or osseous metastases; hoarseness of voice; obstruction of the superior vena cava; jaundice and many others. (4) With non-specific symptoms such as loss of weight and appetite, insomnia, dyspepsia, and so on. (5) With what may be called the humoral (endocrine) or neural concomitants

---

[1] Le Roux, B. T. (1968). The presentation of bronchial carcinoma. *Scott. med. J.* **13**, 31.

of the disease—hypertrophic pulmonary osteoarthropathy; myopathy and neuropathy; Cushing's syndrome and possibly others.

Hypertrophic pulmonary osteoarthropathy and its influence on prognosis is discussed elsewhere; 49 patients presented with this syndrome. Those symptomless patients (192) who presented because of an abnormal routine radiograph are separately grouped and discussed elsewhere in this monograph.

I. PRESENTATION WITH RESPIRATORY SYMPTOMS

1. Cough and Sputum. Of 4,000 patients with bronchial carcinoma, cough was a symptom in 75 per cent, and in 40 per cent cough was severe and one of the primary reasons for seeking medical advice. Cough was, in nearly all instances, productive at some time. In many patients cough was not a new symptom, and was attributed to smoking. In the 40 per cent with severe cough as a presenting symptom, either a chronic cough was ingravescent, or cough was an entirely new symptom, often persisting after one or several acute febrile episodes. Of those who had stopped smoking within weeks of investigation, and who had complained of cough while they still smoked, half found that cough persisted and half that it improved after they had stopped smoking.

2. Haemoptysis. Haemoptysis is known to have been a symptom in 57 per cent of the 4,000 patients with bronchial carcinoma, and in 4 per cent haemoptysis was the only symptom. In 53 per cent haemoptysis was associated with some or all of the other cardinal symptoms of respiratory disease, with one or more febrile illnesses, loss of weight, appetite and energy, and so on. Presentation for investigation in 39 patients (1 per cent) was because of a single haemoptysis. In others with haemoptysis this symptom varied from occasional to daily. The complaint of daily haemoptysis—usually in the form of blood-streaking of the sputum in the early morning—was regarded as typical of bronchial carcinoma as the cause of haemoptysis. Haemoptysis had been a symptom for weeks rather than months in fewer than half the patients with this symptom. Haemoptysis is known to have been tolerated for six to twelve months in 127 patients, including two medical practitioners; for more than a year in 76 patients; for more than two years in 42 patients; for more than three years in 33 patients; for at least five years in two patients and for at least six years in one. Of those who tolerated haemoptysis for more than six months, the symptom occurred daily in more than half. Of those who presented with a single haemoptysis as the only symptom, fewer than half presented within a week of the episode of bleeding, which was small in quantity. In two patients who presented with a radiological abnormality detected after mass radiography there was elicited a history of a single haemoptysis a year earlier. Haemoptysis was the only symptom in four patients who tolerated this for more than two years. Delay in the investigation of haemoptysis in the Thoracic Unit was commonly occasioned by delay in referral for a surgical opinion, rather than delay on the part of the patient in reporting the abnormality.

13

3. Pain. Chest pain was a presenting symptom in 35 per cent of patients, and in very nearly all of these the reason for which medical advice was ultimately sought, although pain was commonly endured for three to four months, and in some patients for as long as eighteen months, before help was enlisted. Acute pleural pain was rare, and rarely endured for more than a few days. Pain was commonly described as an intermittent ache, lasting for hours at a time, worse at night, made worse by posture, and relieved by activity. Severe pain was common in those shown to have invasion of the chest wall, but parietal invasion, vertebral invasion, and costal and vertebral metastases were found in patients who denied pain, and the complaint of pain was not uncommon in patients found to have pulmonary tumours which were successfully managed surgically and in whom pain could not be related to pleural invasion or infection.

4. Dyspnoea. In 45 per cent of patients dyspnoea was an important symptom. In most dyspnoea was of less than a year's duration—in some dyspnoea had become increasingly burdensome for as long as two years. From the records it is not possible to equate the complaint of dyspnoea with diminution in measured respiratory function. Very nearly normal respiratory function figures are recorded for many patients amongst whose more distressing complaints was dyspnoea. Dyspnoea as the only symptom is recorded in only 28 of 4,000 patients, all of whom had a large pleural effusion.

5. Febrile Respiratory Illness. In 22 per cent of patients there was a history either of an acute febrile respiratory illness, often called influenza, from which recovery was slow and incomplete, or of a series of acute febrile illnesses with complete or incomplete recovery between episodes. Cough with purulent sputum, chest pain, dyspnoea and haemoptysis were often features of these acute illnesses, but evanescent features of which little cognisance had been taken during the acute episodes, in fact taken for granted as part of the acute episode. This history, of failure to make an expected recovery from an acute respiratory illness, is accepted as strongly suggestive of the diagnosis of bronchial carcinoma in the same way as is daily haemoptysis.

6. Wheeze. Apart from eight patients who were chronic asthmatics, intermittent wheeze was a presenting symptom in 82 of 4,000 patients (2 per cent). In 17 of these 82 patients wheeze was localised and unilateral. The patients who complained of wheeze were found usually to have a tumour which extended in a main bronchus close to the main carina, and even into the trachea, and as a prognostic feature wheeze, in this group of patients, was, like stridor, often significant of inoperability.

7. Stridor. This, as distinct from intermittent wheeze, was not common—53 patients were recorded as being stridulous at the time of first examination, 29 of them urgently stridulous and in need of therapeutic bronchoscopy, at which tumour was cored from the trachea or both main bronchi in order to establish a more adequate air-way. During the period under discussion two patients were admitted with the diagnosis of bronchial carcinoma, made by referring doctors on the grounds of severe stridor, and at bronchoscopy, in each, the trachea was only red and oedematous, and symptoms disappeared over a period of days with the exhibition of an antibiotic. Before the management of these patients it had not been recognised by the staff of the Unit that acute tracheo-bronchitis in an adult could present with such gross evidence of proximal air-way obstruction.

II. PRESENTATION WITH SYMPTOMS OTHER THAN RESPIRATORY AND RELATED TO DISSEMINATION OF CARCINOMA

1. Of 4,000 patients with bronchial carcinoma, 133 (3·3 per cent) presented not with respiratory symptoms, but to medical out-patient, casualty or neuro-surgical departments with symptoms and signs of intracranial lesions and, in the course of general investigation in most, but after craniotomy in 11, were shown to have *intracranial metastases from bronchial carcinoma.* Some of these patients admitted respiratory symptoms but none had thought it necessary to seek advice for these symptoms. The commonest neurological disturbance leading to admission to hospital was hemiplegia (21 patients); the recent onset of epilepsy prompted referral for advice in 19 patients, in five of whom epilepsy was Jacksonian in type; personality change, or confusional states in 18 patients, speech defects (dysphasia or aphasia) in 15, and cerebellar disturbances in another 15, precipitated admission; 14 patients were investigated for headache alone, and 10 others for headache, vomiting and visual distur-bances; 4 were admitted in coma from increased intracranial pressure; 10 were monoparetic and 7 presented with an isolated cranial nerve palsy.

2. Of 87 patients found to have *osseous metastases* from bronchial car-cinoma as the only evidence at the time of first investigation of dissemination of tumour, presentation in 63 was because of osteocopic pain. Six patients presented because of pain of acute onset in relation to coughing and there was seen radiographically a fracture through a rib metastasis. Two of 31 patients with vertebral metastases presented because of paraplegia and one because of urinary retention. Pathological fracture prompted admission in five patients —of the femur, humerus or clavicle.

3. *Jaundice* was the reason for admission to hospital in four patients who were later shown to have *hepatic metastases* from bronchial carcinoma; one of the patients with jaundice also had ascites, and four other patients not recog-nised as icteric were admitted for the investigation of *ascites* and shown to have hepatic metastases from bronchial carcinoma.

4. Of 4,000 patients with bronchial carcinoma 183 had, at the time of first presentation, the clinical features of *obstruction of the superior vena cava.* Many of these patients had other symptoms such as haemoptysis, cough, dyspnoea and so on, but in most the emergence of the discomfort associated with caval obstruction prompted attendance at hospital.

5. *Dysphagia* was the only presenting complaint in 13 patients; in 47 other patients dysphagia was one of the presenting complaints. In 30 of these

15

60 patients oesophageal displacement and compression, demonstrated at fluoroscopy and confirmed at oesophagoscopy, was the only evidence of tumour spread outwith the lung; in none of this group of 30 was the oesophageal mucosa disrupted and in none was there any reasonable doubt that the primary tumour was pulmonary. In the remaining 30 patients there was evidence of tumour spread other than to mediastinal glands which were responsible for dysphagia, and in these patients there was again no reasonable doubt that the tumour was primarily of the lung. Excluded from the group of 4,000 patients are seven who presented during the period under discussion with dysphagia; in these there was a hilar shadow and squamous carcinoma in the trachea or at the main carina, and in the oesophagus, and four had already developed as oesophago-tracheal fistula. These are excluded because it is not known whether their primary tumour was oesophageal or pulmonary. Where dysphagia is related to malignant disease the tumour responsible for dysphagia is nearly always in the proximal part of the alimentary tract; the only other common causes of malignant dysphagia are mediastinal metastases from primary pulmonary or primary mammary tumours.

6. *Interruption of the left recurrent laryngeal nerve* was the only evidence of extra-pulmonary extension of tumour in 132 patients. Hoarseness of voice was the reason for seeking medical advice in 49 of these 132 patients, and in them this symptom was of a duration which varied from three years to two weeks; in most the complaint was of at least three to four months' duration. In the remaining 83 patients hoarseness of voice was only one of several complaints, which included haemoptysis, dyspnoea and so on, and in some instances the patient did not realise that there was a change in voice.

7. *Metastases in muscle* were encountered in eight patients, and in six of these presentation was because of the appearance of a mass in a muscle—triceps in one, quadriceps in three, calf and rectus abdominis in one each. These six patients denied respiratory symptoms even after a primary pulmonary tumour had been demonstrated by routine radiography in the search for a primary.

8. *Cutaneous or subcutaneous metastases* were the only evidence of dissemination of bronchial carcinoma in 38 patients and in 19 other patients were found in conjunction with additional clinical evidence of spread. In five of these patients presentation was with the complaint of a cutaneous or subcutaneous nodule and these patients denied other symptoms. Cutaneous metastases were always small and the patients were, in some instances, sure that the nodule had been present " for years "; in other instances a nodule had been seen to appear and grow rapidly and, when it had achieved the size of a pea, to cease to grow. Subcutaneous metastases were generally of the size of a cherry when they were clinically recognised. Cutaneous and subcutaneous metastases were more often felt than seen, and the habit of examining the patient's integument by rubbing the palms of the hands over all the skin surfaces is recommended.

9. *Metastases in scars* were found in three patients and, in all, were the reason for presentation. The scar of inguinal hernia repair undertaken 30 years earlier, the scar of empyema drainage 20 years earlier, and the scar of laparotomy, presumably for appendicectomy, 15 years earlier, were the sites of metastases which, in these three patients, constituted the only evidence of dissemination of pulmonary carcinoma, which was recognised after biopsy of the metastasis and chest radiography, in that order.

10. Two men presented with *purpura,* and were found to have splenomegaly; in the course of investigation a pulmonary opacity was seen on chest radiography and sheets of tumour cells were demonstrated in sternal marrow.

11. An *abdominal mass* other than hepatic was found in nine patients who presented with vague abdominal discomfort and without respiratory symptoms. In two of these patients the abdominal mass was *renal,* one of the two had haematuria, and in both the pyelogram was abnormal. The abdominal mass in five patients, shown later to have bronchial carcinoma, was established to be a *supra-renal* metastasis. Supra-renal metastases from bronchial carcinoma are common but are rarely clinically palpable. A pelvic mass in one woman was established after limited laparotomy and biopsy to be an *ovarian* metastasis from bronchial carcinoma. A mobile abdominal mass in a man was found after limited laparotomy and biopsy to be a large metastasis in the greater *omentum.*

12. Presentation in three patients was with a *scalp* metastasis, and other unusual sites of metastasis were the *tongue,* a *tonsil,* the *hard palate,* the *lower alveolus,* a *thumb* and a *second toe*—each of these in one patient. After investigation of these nine patients, in none were these unusual metastases the only evidence of tumour spread, but none presented with symptoms other than those related to the unusual metastasis. The digital metastasis presented in such a way as to make a casualty officer believe that he was dealing with chronic paronychia, and the diagnosis was made only when tumour fungated through a surgical incision some weeks later. The scalp metastases were multiple and limited to the scalp in two patients; in one there was a single scalp metastasis managed surgically in the belief that it was a primary integumental tumour, possibly a sebaceous adenoma.

13. In 37 of 131 patients in whom the primary pulmonary tumour, at the time of first investigation, invaded directly the adjacent chest wall, the tumour was apical and invaded also the brachial plexus and the cervical sympathetic; these patients with *Pancoast's syndrome* presented because of the symptoms associated with parietal invasion. Not all the remaining patients with parietal invasion presented with pain and not all patients who presented with pain had parietal invasion.

III. PRESENTATION WITH NON-SPECIFIC SYMPTOMS

1. Loss of Weight and Appetite. These symptoms, separately or together, were common, but in 8 per cent of cases it was one or both of these general symp-

17

toms which prompted investigation, and in these patients respiratory symptoms were denied, or were of long standing without recent change. In this group of patients the initial radiological investigation undertaken was often a barium meal, and a pulmonary lesion was recognised during routine fluoroscopy of the chest at this examination.

2. Other General Symptoms. In 94 patients complaints were simply those of tiredness and lassitude, and 35 patients had complained to their general practitioners only of feeling generally ill, often vaguely and in a totally non-specific way. Referral of these patients to the Thoracic Unit was in most instances the result of an abnormality having been detected on a chest radiograph made as one of the many routine investigations undertaken in a search for a cause of their non-specific symptoms. These patients are not regarded as having presented because of a radiographic abnormality found on routine or mass miniature films—although in many the initial film was in fact a miniature—because radiography in this group was undertaken because of symptoms, albeit not respiratory symptoms.

3. Dyspepsia. In 21 patients dyspepsia was the only symptom, and in three others dyspepsia was accompanied by persistent vomiting. In this group a pulmonary lesion was recognised at fluoroscopy of the chest during the making of barium studies.

4. Peripheral Venous Thrombosis. Fifteen patients presented without respiratory symptoms of any sort or with respiratory symptoms such as cough or dyspnoea which they had had for so long that they regarded them as normal concomitants of smoking; and with peripheral venous thrombosis, often recurrent, and, in many of the records of this group, called thrombophlebitis migrans. Eleven of these patients were referred from a peripheral vascular disease clinic, to which they had originally been referred by their general practitioner. The tumour was managed surgically in only five of the 15, and two of the five died from pulmonary embolism in early convalescence.

IV. UNUSUAL PRESENTATION

A small number of patients presented either with unusual symptoms probably directly attributable to bronchial carcinoma, or with collateral lesions directly related to bronchial carcinoma.

In seven patients presentation was with carcinomatous myopathy; two patients had as their only complaint insomnia; exfoliative dermatitis in three patients was the only reason for enlisting medical advice; repeated cough syncope brought five patients to hospital, and persistent hiccough two others; four patients sought medical advice because they had noticed the development of finger clubbing—these patients did not have hypertrophic pulmonary osteoarthropathy—and in four other patients admission to hospital was a matter of urgency because of spontaneous pneumothorax, none of the four having had symptoms suggestive of bronchial carcinoma before the acute onset of symptoms; in one the pneumothorax was under tension. In three patients chest radiography was prompted by sudden and otherwise unexplained difficulty in the control of known diabetes mellitus. In one patient a chest radiograph was made because of herpes zoster. Cough in five men was thought likely to jeopardise the success of inguinal herniorrhaphy and chest radiography in these demonstrated abnormalities later shown to be bronchial tumours. Bronchial carcinoma in two patients was detected during investigation of symptoms and signs of acute onset and suggestive of Cushing's syndrome.

OCCUPATION

The occupation of 4,000 patients with bronchial carcinoma is outlined in Table I. The occupation most commonly afflicted in this series is that of coal miner. It is not possible to correlate the incidence of bronchial carcinoma in a particular occupation group with the population at risk in that group, because census figures are not available for 1961. Statisticians of the Scottish Health Department acknowledge that the occupations shown in Table I are representative of the commoner occupations amongst the inhabitants of the South East Region of Scotland; from old census figures the incidence of bronchial carcinoma amongst coal miners may be disproportionately high. Prognosis amongst coal miners is apparently not different from non-miners, unless there is associated pneumoconiosis, when survival rate is increased—an association to be expected if the spread of carcinoma in miner's lungs were impeded by coal dust (Goldman, 1965)[1]. At the present time, no further comment is possible.

SMOKING

Of the 4,000 patients in this series (of whom 403 (10 per cent) were women), 73 per cent are known to have smoked cigarettes. The records are not sufficiently precise to be able to classify this group as heavy, moderate and light smokers. In this group are included those who smoked a pipe or cigars in addition to cigarettes; also included are 28 who had stopped smoking 10 to 20 years before the clinical evidence of bronchial carcinoma was recognised, and 43 men who had stopped smoking three to 10 years before the diagnosis of bronchial carcinoma was made.

Of the 4,000 patients, 3 per cent smoked only a pipe, and 4 per cent—62 women and 99 men—claimed never to have smoked. Amongst the women in the series, therefore, 15 per cent claimed never to have smoked. During the last five to six years there has emerged a noticeable reluctance amongst patients to admit that they smoked, and it is now commonplace for patients when asked the question " Do you smoke?" to answer, quite honestly, in the negative, on the grounds that they had stopped smoking with the onset of symptoms, or with the finding of an abnormality on a chest radiograph, or even the day before interrogation. On the other hand, those who denied smoking in the circumstances outlined above will admit to having smoked if properly and persistently

[1] Goldman, K. P. (1965). Prognosis of coal-miners with cancer of the lung. *Thorax*, **20**, 170.

TABLE I

Occupation

Occupation	No. involved from 4,000	Per cent	Comments
Miners	624	15·6	Nearly all coal miners, a few stone and limestone workers, etc.
Transport workers	391	9·8	Railways, bus services, van drivers, long and short haul lorry drivers, taxi drivers, chauffeurs.
Heavy industry	367	9·2	Sheet metal workers, fitters and turners, paper makers, ammunition workers, bricklayers, boiler makers, iron moulders, etc.
Unskilled labourers	299	7·5	
Professions	249	6·2	Civil servants, doctors, bankers, veterinary surgeons, teachers, journalists, lawyers, dentists, chemists, executives, laboratory technicians, etc.
Shopkeepers	229	5·7	Grocers, tailors, newsagents and tobacconists, butchers, storemen.
Crafts & Trades	227	5·7	Gold and silversmiths, joiners, painters, blacksmiths, cobblers, printers, polishers, etc.
Engineers	185	4·6	Mining, electrical, mechanical, civil, etc.
Ships & Shipping	183	4·6	
Outdoor workers	179	4·5	Farmers, farmhands, shepherds, poultry workers, water bailiffs, greenkeepers, groundsmen, gardeners, nurserymen, etc.
Hoteliers & brewery workers	156	3·9	Hoteliers, barmen, coopers, brewery labourers.
Salesmen	114	2·9	Insurance, shops, commercial travellers, etc.
Fisheries	91	2·3	
Bakers & confectioners	89	2·2	
Watchmen	88	2·2	Nearly all elderly and retired from other occupations.
Hosiery & tweed-mill workers	79	2	
Others	450	Each group less than 2	Post and telegraphs, army, vagrants, housewives, tax inspectors, bookmakers, billposters, Forth Rail Bridge painters, dustmen, flour-millers, potato merchants, garage proprietors, scrap-metal merchants, undertakers, firemen, policemen, linoleum workers, unknown.

Where patients were retired at the time of admission, their previous occupations were recorded, and where a patient had been occupied in different ways, the period of longest occupation was recorded.

interrogated. The 4 per cent accepted as non-smokers includes only those regarding whose non-smoking habits there is no reasonable doubt. The tumour in the 161 non-smokers was in 58 squamous, in 79 undifferentiated, in 13 an adenocarcinoma and in 11 of unknown histology.

The smoking habits of 20 per cent of the 4,000 patients are not recorded. This omission is probably significant of a similar failure in all other aspects of the anamneses and a sound argument in favour of demanding from rotational junior staff who interrogate patients the completion of a detailed pro forma rather than the recording of answers to those variable questions which they may remember to ask.

III

Investigation

APART from a small number of patients too ill at the time of admission to withstand routine investigation, or who died before investigation could be completed, all patients were submitted to a routine series of investigations. History and clinical examination were recorded in detail, although, from the records, there was clearly considerable variation in the degree of detail. For example, 60 per cent of patients are recorded as having clubbed fingers, but in the first 2,000 patients 75 per cent had clubbed fingers, and in the second 2,000 only 46 per cent—it is unlikely that the two groups would vary over such a wide range. Routine chest radiographs were made, and all patients well enough to go to the X-ray Department were examined behind the X-ray screen, primarily to search for evidence of phrenic paresis and displacement of the barium-filled oesophagus. Tomograms and other special films were made in circumstances in which they were believed necessary, for diagnostic or record purposes. Bronchoscopy was a routine, and biopsies were made from visible tumours. In 2,320 patients bronchoscopy established unequivocally the diagnosis of bronchial carcinoma—that is, the tumours were central in 58 per cent of patients. In 1,680 patients (42 per cent), the appearances at bronchoscopy were normal, or there was only bronchial compression or distortion without mucosal abnormality, and these patients are recorded as having tumours of peripheral type. At no stage in the period under discussion was bronchography regarded as contributory to the establishment of the diagnosis of bronchial carcinoma. Pleural effusion was investigated by thoracentesis, examination of the pleural liquid, replacement of the effusion with air, thoracoscopy, and pleural biopsy under vision. Biopsy of cervical lymph nodes was made where glands were palpable, and not as a routine. Biopsy was made from other easily accessible metastases—in skin, subcutaneous and other soft tissues, and in muscle. Sputum was examined for tumour cells routinely after 1955, in an attempt to evaluate the place of this examination as part of standard practice. Symptoms such as bone pain, haematuria, and so on, were investigated appropriately; a search was not made routinely for possible silent metastases, by radiographic skeletal surveys, by routine pyelography, or similar techniques. Special examinations, such as pneumomediastinography (Símeček and Holeb, 1961)[1], were occasionally undertaken in unusual circumstances,

[1] Símeček, C. & Holeb, E. (1961). Pneumomediastinography in carcinoma of the lung. *Thorax*, **16**, 65.

but were also never a part of the routine. Respiratory function—in particular the forced expiratory volume—was measured in patients in whom surgical management was contemplated, but was rarely found more informative than an assessment of function on the ground of exercise tolerance. An electrocardiogram was made pre-operatively in all patients over the age of 40 years. Latterly, all routine pre-operative chest radiographs, made on the day before operation, were antero-posterior films made with portable radiographic apparatus with the patient in bed, to provide a more precise base-line against which to judge post-operative films. A search for tubercle bacilli was made on specimens of sputum from all patients.

With regard to the radiographic appearances of bronchial carcinoma, postero-anterior and appropriate lateral radiographs were normal in three of 4,000 patients with bronchial carcinoma—normal on repeated films, and normal to a number of individual experts. In these three patients presentation was with haemoptysis in all, in one associated with wheeze. The tumours were visible at bronchoscopy in a main bronchus in all, and also in the trachea in one.

Tuberculous pulmonary cavitation was a radiographically recognised concomitant of bronchial carcinoma in 43 patients—in 15 of these tuberculous cavities were bilateral. Tubercle bacilli were found in the sputum from 69 patients, 23 of whom were known to have pulmonary tuberculosis and who were referred from sanatoria. The radiographic changes of pneumoconiosis were commonplace; in 33 patients the radiographic features of progressive massive fibrosis were recognised and in three patients radiographic features compatible with the diagnosis of Caplan's syndrome were recorded. Pleural effusion was recorded as an accompaniment of bronchial carcinoma in 480 patients. Bullous emphysema was a common accompaniment of bronchial carcinoma in older patients, while obstructive emphysema the consequence of bronchial carcinoma was recognised in only 15 patients. The incidence of lymphangitis carcinomatosa and of pulmono-pulmonary metastases is discussed elsewhere.

In 279 (7 per cent) of 4,000 patients with bronchial carcinoma there were related cardiovascular abnormalities. The commonest single abnormality was systemic hypertension—in 75 patients the diastolic blood pressure was consistently higher than 110 mm. Hg, and the systolic pressure was usually above 200 mm. Hg, and there was electrocardiographic evidence of left ventricular hypertrophy. There was a previous history of myocardial infarction in 59 other patients, and in 54 patients there was a history of angina pectoris. At the time of admission 37 patients were in congestive cardiac failure; in 42 other patients the atrial rhythm was that of fibrillation and in seven others that of flutter. Two patients had mitral stenosis; two other patients had mitral and aortic stenosis; the last of this group had an aneurysm of the innominate artery.

In 27 of this group of 279 patients, myocardial or vascular disease was accepted as the only contra-indication to surgical management of bronchial carcinoma; in 105 patients, in addition to a cardiovascular abnormality, there was evidence of dissemination of tumour which precluded surgical management. In 147 patients—75 with systemic hypertension, 43 with a history of myocardial infarction, and 29 with a history of angina—bronchial carcinoma was managed surgically, and in 103 of these 147 patients a resection was achieved. Operative mortality amongst the 44 patients with cardiovascular disease and bronchial carcinoma in whom only an exploration was made was 25 per cent (11 patients)—four times the operative mortality for exploration without resection in the series as a whole—but only four of the 11 patients who died did so unequivocally from a cardiovascular cause. Operative mortality amongst the 103 patients with bronchial carcinoma and cardiovascular disease submitted either to lobectomy or to pneumonectomy was 35 per cent—again four times that of pneumonectomy or lobectomy in the series as a whole, irrespective of age at the time of the resection. Thirty-six patients with bronchial carcinoma and cardiovascular disease died in convalescence after pulmonary resection, and half of those who died, died from an acute cardiovascular episode—myocardial infarction, or congestive cardiac failure.

Of 4,000 patients with bronchial carcinoma, 17 had severe rheumatoid arthritis; 10 of these were coal miners, and in three there were the radiographic appearances accepted as those of Caplan's syndrome, which, in one of the three, obscured the diagnosis of bronchial carcinoma for some considerable time. Pulmonary tuberculosis was an accompaniment of bronchial carcinoma in 69 patients. Ankylosing spondylitis in five patients, chronic glomerulo-nephritis in three and Parkinson's disease in another three were found to accompany bronchial carcinoma; and acromegaly, syringomyelia and multiple sclerosis were concomitants of bronchial carcinoma—each in one patient.

IV

The Influence of Predominant Cell Type on Management and Prognosis[1]

SUMMARY

Of 4,000 patients with bronchial carcinoma, the histology of the tumour was known in all but 5·8 per cent; nearly 48 per cent of tumours were squamous; 40 per cent were undifferentiated; 5 per cent were adenocarcinomata; in 17 patients the tumour was an alveolar cell carcinoma; in 56 patients submitted to exploratory thoracotomy the histology of the tumour was mixed. Squamous tumours were more often operable than were undifferentiated tumours. More than half the patients with adenocarcinoma and alveolar cell carcinoma were surgically managed.

Mediastinal glandular metastases from squamous or undifferentiated carcinoma demonstrated after pulmonary resection, did not preclude long survival. More patients younger than 40 years managed by pneumonectomy had undifferentiated than had squamous tumours; squamous tumours were nearly three times more common in those managed by pneumonectomy over the age of 40 years. Operative mortality after pneumonectomy was relatively highest in those with an adenocarcinoma. There was evidence at necropsy of distant spread in more than 80 per cent of patients who died in the early post-operative period after pneumonectomy. The death rate in those submitted to pneumonectomy for undifferentiated carcinoma was more rapid in the first three post-operative years than in those submitted to pneumonectomy for squamous carcinoma. One in every three patients who died from metastases in the first two years after pneumonectomy died with cerebral metastases.

Lobectomy in 65 per cent of patients was for squamous carcinoma, and was only slightly more common for undifferentiated carcinoma (18 per cent) than for adenocarcinoma (15 per cent). The mortality from metastases after lobectomy for adenocarcinoma was disproportionately high in the second year after resection. Long survival after lobectomy for squamous or undifferentiated carcinoma with glandular metastases was not uncommon.

Segmental resection in a small number of patients, most with squamous or adenocarcinoma, was followed by long survival in more than a quarter.

Bronchial carcinoma in patients who presented without symptoms and with an abnormal routine chest radiograph, made for unrelated purpose, was most often squamous, peripheral in type, and of small size. In this group the rate of resectability and of long survival was high and operative mortality was small.

A third of the patients with bronchial carcinoma, who denied ever having smoked, had squamous tumours. The incidence of adenocarcinoma in women, and those with hypertrophic pulmonary osteoarthropathy, was significantly higher. Many patients in whom bronchial adenocarcinoma was managed surgically died with cerebral metastases.

[1] Le Roux, B. T. (1968). The influence of predominant cell type on the management and prognosis of bronchial carcinoma. *Scott. med. J.*, **13**, 84.

The incidence of resectability with long survival in a small group of patients with alveolar cell carcinoma was surprisingly high.

Lymphangitis carcinomatosa and interruption of the left recurrent laryngeal nerve were found disproportionately often with squamous carcinoma. Osseous metastases from adenocarcinoma were rare and pleural metastases common. Obstruction of the superior vena cava was caused disproportionately often by undifferentiated tumours.

THE purpose here is to review the histology of the tumours in 4,000 patients with bronchial carcinoma and to relate predominant histological type to management and prognosis. From scrutiny of the literature[1, 2, 3] there is clearly variability over a wide range in the prognostic significance attributed to different cell types and in the interpretation of the same histological material by different histologists. Cell type should not influence the selection of patients for surgical management.

In 232 patients (5·8 per cent) a histological diagnosis was never established, but in these patients the diagnosis of bronchial carcinoma was beyond reasonable doubt. In 3,768 patients the histological diagnosis was achieved, and the incidence of the histological types is shown in Table II. The group of

TABLE II

Bronchial Carcinoma

4,000 Patients

Histology

Squamous	1,901	(47·5%)
Undifferentiated	1,592	(39·8%)
Adenocarcinoma	202	(5·1%)
Alveolar cell carcinoma	17	(0·4%)
Mixed	56	(1·4%)
Unknown	232	(5·8%)
Total	4,000	

undifferentiated tumours includes " anaplastic " and " oat cell " carcinoma. A number of pathologists examined biopsy and operative specimens, and some did not use the term " oat cell " tumour; it has, therefore, been necessary to group " oat cell " carcinomas with the other undifferentiated tumours. More than half the tumours with known histology were squamous—the ratio of squamous to undifferentiated tumours was about 5 to 4. Adenocarcinoma was uncommon and comprised only 5 per cent of the series; alveolar cell carcinoma (0·4 per cent of the series) was rare. In 56 patients managed

[1] Siddons, A. H. M. (1962). Cell type in the choice of cases of carcinoma of the bronchus for surgery. *Thorax*, 17, 308.
[2] Taylor, A. B., Shinton, N. K. & Waterhouse, J. A. H. (1963). Histology of bronchial carcinoma in relation to prognosis. *Thorax*, 18, 178.
[3] Goldman, K.P. (1965). Histology of lung cancer in relation to prognosis. *Thorax*, 20, 298.

surgically, the histology of a biopsy made at bronchoscopy was different from the histology of the operative specimen or of glands in the mediastinum.

Management of 4,000 patients with bronchial carcinoma is outlined in Table III, and in Table IV the histology of the tumour in the 1,783 patients

TABLE III

Bronchial Carcinoma

Management in 4,000 Patients

Surgical 1,783 (44·6%)	Pneumonectomy	977
	Lobectomy	470
	Segmental resection	17
	Exploratory thoracotomy only	319
Non-surgical	Because of clinical, radiographic, fluoroscopic or bronchoscopic evidence of metastases	1,834 (45·9%)
2,217 (55·4%)	Because of evidence other than metastatic of unsuitability for surgical management	383 (9·5%)
4,000		4,000

TABLE IV

Bronchial Carcinoma

4,000 Patients

Histology Related to Surgical Management

	Squamous	Undif.	Adeno.	Alveolar	Mixed
Exploration only (319)	163	139	15	—	2
Pneumonectomy (977)	587	311	35	5	39
Lobectomy (470)	292	85	71	7	15
Segmental resection (17)	12	1	4	—	—
Total (1,783)	1,054	536	125	12	56

managed surgically is shown. While the ratio of squamous tumours to undifferentiated tumours in the series as a whole was about 5 to 4, the ratio of squamous to undifferentiated tumours in all those managed surgically was nearly 2 to 1 and in those managed by lobectomy nearly 4 to 1. More than half the total number of patients with an adenocarcinoma who were regarded as suitable candidates for an operation had a tumour which was manageable by lobectomy. Of the small total number of patients (17) with an alveolar cell tumour, 12 were surgically manageable.

Management in patients with squamous tumours is histographically compared with management in patients with undifferentiated tumours in Figure 1. The total of 307 patients managed by lobectomy for squamous carcinoma includes 15 with tumours of mixed histology with a predominantly squamous pattern. Of the undifferentiated tumours 66 per cent were unsuitable for any form of surgical management, in comparison with only 44 per cent of squamous tumours. Only 5 per cent of undifferentiated tumours were suitable for management by lobectomy, whereas 16 per cent of patients with squamous tumours were suitable for this relatively limited operation.

EXPLORATION AT THORACOTOMY WITHOUT RESECTION

Thoracotomy with a view to resection of pulmonary carcinoma was undertaken in 319 patients (8 per cent) in whom the tumour was found either to be technically irresectable or to be associated with evidence of dissemination of tumour which made pulmonary resection pointless. Of the 319 patients 26 were women and 293 were men, a male:female ratio of 11 to 1. Death could be related more or less directly to operation in 20 patients, all of them men—an operative mortality of 6 per cent. In 197 patients histological confirmation of the diagnosis of bronchial carcinoma had been obtained before thoracotomy by biopsy made at bronchoscopy—these patients had central tumours. The bronchoscopic appearances in 122 patients with tumours of peripheral type were normal. In 163 patients the tumour was squamous, and in 139 undifferentiated (in 28 of these called "oat cell"). In 15 patients the tumour was

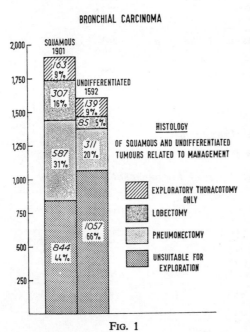

FIG. 1

an adenocarcinoma; in two patients with central tumours the tumour was typed histologically as squamous on the ground of the bronchoscopic biopsy, and the biopsy made at operation was interpreted as an adenocarcinoma in one, and an "oat cell" carcinoma in the other. The ratio of undifferentiated to squamous carcinoma in this group of 319 patients is nearly 9 to 10—a disproportionately high incidence of undifferentiated tumours as compared both with the series as a whole and with those submitted to exploratory thoracotomy.

28

MANAGEMENT BY PNEUMONECTOMY

Bronchial carcinoma in 977 patients (24 per cent) was managed by pneumonectomy—on the right in 462 and on the left in 515. In 290 patients the tumour was peripheral in type and in these the appearances at bronchoscopy were normal. In this group the tumours were most commonly located in an upper lobe and more often in the left upper lobe. In 687 patients the tumour was central in type, and histological confirmation of the diagnosis of bronchial carcinoma was obtained in this group of patients by biopsy at bronchoscopy. Central tumours were as common in the upper as in the lower lobes, and on the right as on the left. The histological range in this group of 977 pneumonectomies is shown in Tables V-IX. Squamous tumours were the most common (587); there were 311 undifferentiated tumours and only 35 adenocarcinomata; in five the tumour was an alveolar cell carcinoma, and in 39 patients the histological diagnosis from biopsy at bronchoscopy differed from the operative specimen or the mediastinal glands (Table X).

TABLE V

Pneumonectomy (977 Patients)

Histology—All Cases

	No. of cases	*No. in previous column with positive glands*
Squamous	587	196 (33%)
Undifferentiated	311	171 (55%)
Adenocarcinoma	35	13 (37%)
Alveolar	5	4
Mixed	39	16
Total	977	400 (41%)

TABLE VI

Pneumonectomy

Histology—Peripheral Tumours

	No. of cases	*No. in previous column with positive glands*
Squamous	152	57 (37%)
Undifferentiated	109	64 (58%)
Adenocarcinoma	21	8
Alveolar	5	4
Mixed	3	3
Total	290	136 (46%)

29

TABLE VII

Pneumonectomy

Squamous Carcinoma (587 Patients)

Histology in Relation to Age

MALE			FEMALE		
Half-Decade	*No. of Patients*	*No. with +ve glands*	*Half-Decade*	*No. of Patients*	*No. with +ve glands*
Youngest 29 yrs.	1	—			
35-39	7	2			
40-44	24	8	40-44	2	—
45-49	58	21	45-49	1	1
50-54	97	32	50-54	1	—
55-59	156	54	55-59	5	2
60-64	112	40	60-64	5	—
65-69	74	24	65-69	7	2
70-74	32	7	70-74	1	—
75-79	4	3			
Total	565	191		22	5

Total 587 of which glands were positive in 196. 152 tumours were peripheral and of these glands were positive in 57.

TABLE VIII

Pneumonectomy

Histology in Relation to Age

Undifferentiated Carcinoma (311 Patients)

MALE			FEMALE		
Half-Decade	*No. of Patients*	*No. with +ve glands*	*Half-Decade*	*No. of Patients*	*No. with +ve glands*
Youngest 25 & 28 (oat)	2	2	Youngest 19, 22 & 25 (oat)	3	2
30-34	5	4	30-34	1	1
35-39	8	5	35-39	2	—
40-44	14	10	40-44	1	—
45-49	26	7	45-49	4	—
50-54	45	26	50-54	7	5
55-59	65	36	55-59	8	3
60-64	56	32	60-64	10	4
65-69	42	26	65-69	4	3
70-74	7	4	70-74	1	1
Total	270	152		41	19

Total 311 of which glands were positive in 171. 109 tumours were peripheral and of these glands were positive in 64. Of 311 tumours 27 were called oat-cell, and in these glands were positive in 18.

TABLE IX

Pneumonectomy

Histology in Relation to Age

Adenocarcinoma (35 Patients)

MALE			FEMALE		
Half-Decade	No. of Patients	No. with +ve glands	Half-Decade	No. of Patients	No. with +ve glands
			40-44	1	1
45-49	4	1			
50-54	4	1	50-54	1	—
55-59	8	4			
60-64	5	4	60-64	1	—
65-69	8	2			
70-74	2	—	70-74	1	—
Total	31	12		4	1

Total 35 of which glands were positive in 13. 21 tumours were peripheral and of these glands were positive in 8.

ALVEOLAR CARCINOMA

Men	Ages	Positive Glands
4	61/62/63/67	3
Women		
1	65	1
—		—
5 All peripheral		4

TABLE X

Pneumonectomy

Histology in Relation to Age

Mixed Histology

No. of Cases	Sex		Ages	B'scopic Biopsy	Operative Specimen	Glands
	Male	Female				
2	2	—	59/73	Squamous	Adenocarcinoma	—
2	2	—	53/68 (P)	—	Squamous	Adenocarcinoma
1	1	—	58 (P)	—	,,	Undif.
1	1	—	63	Alveolar	Adenocarcinoma	Adenocarcinoma
2	2	—	59/64	Undif.	,,	—
1	1	—	58 (P)	—	,,	Undif.
2	2	—	48/59	Squamous	Oat cell	—
1	1	—	61	Oat cell	Squamous	Squamous
11	11	—	39/50/52/56/ 57/58/58/59/ 61/66/67	Undif.	,,	—
7	5	2	49/62/64/65/ 69/69/71	,,	,,	Squamous
6	5	1	24/44/55/55/ 63/66	Squamous	Undif.	—
2	2	—	61/63	,,	,,	Undif.
1	1	—	47	,,	Squamous	,,
39	36	3				

3 peripheral tumours indicated as (P)

Mediastinal glands were invaded in 41 per cent of patients in whom pneumonectomy was undertaken—in 33 per cent with squamous tumours, 55 per cent with undifferentiated tumours, more than a third of the 35 patients with adenocarcinoma, four of the five with alveolar cell tumours, and in nearly half of those in whom the cell type was mixed. The incidence of lymph glandular metastases was higher for all histological types in patients submitted to pneumonectomy for peripheral tumours—46 per cent overall, 37 per cent with squamous tumours, and 58 per cent with undifferentiated tumours. The relationship between the histological type of the tumours and the age of the patient is shown in Figure 2. Between the ages of 45 and 70 years, for any half decade, squamous tumours occurred with a frequency a little less than three times that of undifferentiated tumours; under the age of 40 years, squamous tumours, amongst a small total number of patients, were less common than undifferentiated tumours; over the age of 70 years, again amongst only a small total number of patients, five in every six were squamous.

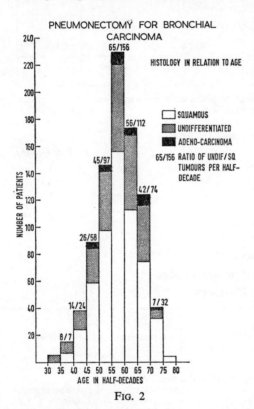

FIG. 2

Eight women and 113 men died as a direct consequence of pneumonectomy for bronchial carcinoma —an overall operative mortality of 12 per cent. The tumour was squamous in 72 of those who died as the consequence of pneumonectomy, undifferentiated in 37, mixed in five and an adenocarcinoma in seven —an operative mortality relatively highest in those with adenocarcinoma. The three common causes of death in the post-operative period after pneumonectomy were respiratory infection, coronary thrombosis and pulmonary embolism. Unsuspected hepatic metastases were found in 17 of 121 patients who died in convalescence after pneumonectomy. Supra-renal metastases were found in nine other patients; small cerebral metastases were found in 11 patients—nine of these had hepatic or supra-renal metastases also. Glandular spread outwith the area cleared of glands at pneumonectomy was found in 42 patients who did not have other evidence of spread. Only 21 of 121 patients who died after pneumonectomy were found not to have evidence of tumour spread—necropsy could not be undertaken in 10 patients.

Of the 786 patients who survived pneumonectomy for bronchial carcinoma, 77 have died from causes not related to recurrence of the tumour. The tumour in 54 of these patients had been squamous, in 16 undifferentiated, in four an adenocarcinoma, in one an alveolar cell carcinoma, and in two the broncho-scopic biopsy differed in histological appearance from the operative specimen. Five of these 77 patients died from other tumours—all adenocarcinomata, one of the rectum, one of the colon, one at the pylorus, one in the body of the stomach and one at the oesophago-gastric junction—the pulmonary tumours in four having been squamous and in one undifferentiated. The second tumour was recognised three to nine years after pneumonectomy; in none was surgical management of the second tumour undertaken; all were over 55 years at the time of pneumonectomy and one was 70 years of age. In this group of 77 patients there was evidence, by necropsy, of absence of tumour recurrence or metastases in 59; in the remainder—all of whom died more than three years after pneumonectomy—there was no clinical evidence of recurrence at the time of death, and on a chest radiograph, made in all within seven months of death, the appearances were normal after pneumonectomy. The causes of death in the group of 77 patients include coronary thrombosis, acute coronary artery insufficiency compli-cating effort angina, cor pulmonale,

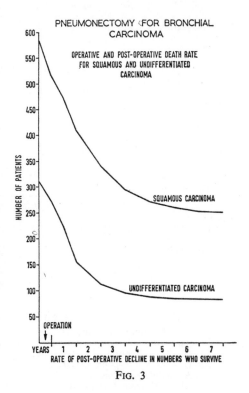

PNEUMONECTOMY FOR BRONCHIAL CARCINOMA

OPERATIVE AND POST-OPERATIVE DEATH RATE FOR SQUAMOUS AND UNDIFFERENTIATED CARCINOMA

SQUAMOUS CARCINOMA

UNDIFFERENTIATED CARCINOMA

OPERATION

YEARS

RATE OF POST-OPERATIVE DECLINE IN NUMBERS WHO SURVIVE

FIG. 3

congestive cardiac failure, pulmonary infection, a second primary tumour in the group of five mentioned above; and rare causes such as dissecting aortic aneurysm, miliary tuberculosis, cerebral vascular accident, and so on. Medias-tinal glandular metastases had been histologically proven at the time of pneumonectomy in 17 patients with squamous tumours and in 7 with un-differentiated tumours in this group of 77 patients.

Of the 977 patients managed by pneumonectomy 510 have died from metastases—107 within six months of operation, a further 141 within a year of resection, 119 more in the second year after resection, and the remainder 3 to 11 years after resection. In Table XI are shown the results of pneumonectomy for bronchial carcinoma in relation to the histological type of the resected tumour. All but two of the 35 patients with adenocarcinoma had died within five years of operation—whether or not glands were invaded at the time of

33

Table XI

Pneumonectomy

Results of Resection

		Histology									
		Sq.	*Sq.+*	*U.*	*U.+*	*Ad.*	*Ad.+*	*Alv.*	*Mixed*	*Total*	
	Operative deaths	52	20	17	20	5	2	—	5	121	
	Non-metastatic deaths	47	6	12	3	3	1	1	4	77	
Deaths from Metastases	Within 6 mths. of op.	14	28	17	35	4	3	1	5	107	510
	6-12 mths. after op.	24	39	29	38	4	1	—	6	141	
	1-2 yrs. after op.	31	35	17	24	2	4	—	6	119	
	2-3 ,, ,, ,,	25	24	7	10	—	1	—	3	70	
	3-4 ,, ,, ,,	16	7	3	5	2	—	—	2	35	
	4-5 ,, ,, ,,	6	4	2	3	—	1	—	1	17	
	5-6 ,, ,, ,,	7	2	—	—	—	—	—	—	9	
	6-7 ,, ,, ,,	2	1	—	—	—	—	—	1	4	
	7-8 ,, ,, ,,	1	—	3	—	—	—	—	1	5	
	9-10 ,, ,, ,,	1	—	—	—	—	—	—	—	1	
	11-12 ,, ,, ,,	2	—	—	—	—	—	—	—	2	
		228	166	107	138	20	13	2	34	708	
	Alive with metastases	18	2	—	10	—	—	—	1	31	
	Alive and well	145	28	33	23	2	—	3+	4	238	
		391	196	140	171	22	13	5	39	977	
		587		311		35					

+ = with glandular metastases.

Sq. = Squamous Carcinoma.
Sq. + = Squamous Carcinoma with Glandular Metastases.
U. = Undifferentiated Carcinoma.
U. + = Undifferentiated Carcinoma with Glandular Metastases.
Ad. = Adenocarcinoma.
Alv. = Alveolar Carcinoma.

pneumonectomy. The death rates, including operative mortality, for squamous and undifferentiated carcinoma, in the first three years after pneumonectomy are shown in Figure 3. At the end of three years 50 per cent of the total number of patients submitted to pneumonectomy, and 57 per cent of those who survived pneumonectomy for squamous carcinoma were alive; in comparison, only 31 per cent of the total number of patients submitted to pneumonectomy and 35 per cent of those who survived pneumonectomy for undifferentiated carcinoma were alive. In the fourth and subsequent years the death rates from metastases or recurrence after pneumonectomy for either squamous or undifferentiated carcinoma were similar and less rapid, but death from metastases or recurrence occurred even 12 years after pneumonectomy. One in every 3 of 367 patients who died from metastases within two years of pneumonectomy

TABLE XII

Pneumonectomy

Histology of Resected Tumours in Those Alive and Well

Period of survival	Histology								
	Sq.	Sq.+	U.	U.+	Ad.	Ad.+	Alv.	Mixed	Total
2-3 yrs.	14	—	5	5	—	—	1+	—	25
3-4 yrs.	18	1	2	4	—	—	1+	—	26
4-5 yrs.	18	3	1	8	—	—	—	—	30
5-6 yrs.	7	3	—	2	—	—	—	—	12
6-7 yrs.	6	2	1	1	—	—	—	—	10
7-8 yrs.	4	1	1	—	—	—	1+	—	7
8-9 yrs	9	2	1	2	—	—	—	—	14
9-10 yrs.	8	3	2	—	—	—	—	2	15
10-11 yrs.	15	2	1	—	—	—	—	—	18
11-12 yrs.	8	3	1	—	—	—	—	1	13
12-13 yrs.	10	3	3	—	—	—	—	—	16
13-14 yrs.	13	2	2	—	—	—	—	—	17
14-15 yrs.	11	1	6	—	—	—	—	1	19
15-16 yrs.	4	2	3	1	—	—	—	—	10
16-17 yrs.	—	—	4	—	2	—	—	—	6
Total	145	28	33	23	2	—	3	4	238

173   56

+ =with glandular metastases.

died with cerebral metastases as the only clinical evidence of tumour dissemination.

At the time when the survey was completed, 31 patients were alive after pneumonectomy, but had clinical or radiological evidence of metastases.

In Table XII the histology of the resected tumour is related to survival time in the 238 patients known to be alive and well and without clinically or radiographically recognised metastases at the time of completing this survey. The six who survived longest were submitted to pneumonectomy more than 16 years ago—two for adenocarcinoma (these are the only two patients alive after pneumonectomy for adenocarcinoma, and both would now have been managed by lobectomy) and four for undifferentiated carcinoma. Of those alive, 25 per cent had glandular metastases at the time of pneumonectomy.

The outcome of surgical management by pneumonectomy of 35 patients with adenocarcinoma, and a further eight patients with mixed tumours which included adenocarcinoma, can be summarised: seven died as the direct consequence of operation; five died one to eight years after operation, from causes other than recurrence of tumour; 15 died with cerebral metastases, 13 of them within a year of operation; 13 died from tumour recurrence or metastases other than cerebral, most more than a year after operation; and three are alive, two 16 years after pneumonectomy and one in whom the histological appearances of the bronchoscopic biopsy were those of undifferentiated carcinoma and the operative specimen those of adenocarcinoma, 14 years after pneumonectomy.

Some of those at present alive more than two but less than five years after pneumonectomy will almost certainly die from metastases, as will some of those alive more than five years after pneumonectomy and apparently well at the present time. But of 977 patients submitted to pneumonectomy for carcinoma 238 (24 per cent) were alive more than two years after pneumonectomy without clinical or radiographic evidence of metastases. Of 788 patients submitted to pneumonectomy more than five years ago 157 (20 per cent) were alive and well, without evidence of metastases.

MANAGEMENT BY LOBECTOMY

Bronchial carcinoma in 470 patients (12 per cent) was managed by lobectomy—by the resection of a single lobe in 318; by the resection of two lobes in 91 patients; and by the resection of a lobe or two lobes with part of the stem bronchus (" sleeve resection ") in 61 patients. Where a single lobe was resected the tumour was peripheral in five of every six resections undertaken. Where two lobes were resected, or a sleeve resection was undertaken, the tumour was more commonly central than peripheral. The histological range in this group of 470 lobectomies is shown in Tables XIII and XIV. Squamous

TABLE XIII

Lobectomy

Histology

	Male	Female	Total	Positive glands
Squamous	296	11	307	83
Undifferentiated	73	12	85	25
Adenocarcinoma	56	15	71	9
Alveolar	6	1	7	1
Total	431	39	470	118

TABLE XIV

Mixed Histology (Included in Table XIII under Squamous)

No. of cases	B'scopic biopsy	Operative specimen	Glands
4	Undifferentiated	Squamous	—
4	Squamous	Undifferentiated	Squamous
2	Squamous	Oat	Oat
2	Squamous	Adenocarcinoma	Alveolar
3	Squamous	Squamous	Undifferentiated
15			

TABLE XV

Lobectomy

Results of Resection

	Sex		Histology				
	Male	Female	Sq.	U.	Ad.	Alv.	Total
Operative death	33	2	24	7	3	1	35
Non-metastatic death	35	2	28	6	3	—	37
Within 6 mths. of op.	12	2	6	7	1	—	14
6-12 mths. after op.	40	3	27	9	6	1	43
1-2 yrs. after op.	53	2	29	12	14	—	55
2-3 ,, ,, ,,	13	2	13	1	1	—	15
3-4 ,, ,, ,,	15	2	14	—	3	—	17
4-5 ,, ,, ,,	11	—	6	1	4	—	11
5-6 ,, ,, ,,	6	—	5	1	—	—	6
6-7 ,, ,, ,,	2	—	2	—	—	—	2
7-8 ,, ,, ,,	4	—	4	—	—	—	4
8-9 ,, ,, ,,	4	—	4	—	—	—	4
Alive with metastases	6	1	5	—	1	1	7
	234	16	167	44	36	3	250
Alive and well	197	23	140	41	35	4	220
	431	39	307	85	71	7	470

Deaths from Metastases — 171

tumours were the most common (65 per cent); undifferentiated tumours (18 per cent) and adenocarcinomata (15 per cent) were of nearly equal frequency, and the number of undifferentiated tumours managed by lobectomy is very much smaller than the number found irresectable and the number managed by pneumonectomy. Where the cell type found at bronchoscopic biopsy differed from that of the operative specimen or mediastinal glands, one of the cell types was, in all the 15 instances, of squamous carcinoma. Two women and 33 men died as the direct consequence of operation—an operative mortality of 7 per cent. None of the patients submitted to " sleeve resection " died. The two common causes of post-operative death were pulmonary embolism, and pulmonary infection with pulmonary insufficiency.

Of those who survived operation, 37 patients have died from causes not related to tumour recurrence. The causes were similar to those listed in the section devoted to pneumonectomy. In Table XV are shown the results of resection in relation to the histological type of the resected tumour. Of the 470 patients in whom bronchial carcinoma was managed by lobectomy, 171 have died from metastases—14 within six months of resection, a further 43 within a year of resection, 55 more in the second year after resection, and the remainder three to nine years after resection. The mortality from metastases from adeno-carcinomas seems disproportionately high in the second year after resection.

TABLE XVI

Lobectomy

Histology of Resected Tumours in Those Alive and Well

Period of survival	Histology						
	Sq.	Sq.+	U.	U.+	Ad.	Alv.	Total
2-3 yrs.	16	6	5	3	6	—	36
3-4 yrs.	12	4	4	2	3	1	26
4-5 yrs.	13	2	2	1	5	1	24
5-6 yrs.	12	3	4	2	3	—	24
6-7 yrs.	15	2	3	1	6	1	28
7-8 yrs.	6	2	3	2	3	1	17
8-9 yrs.	10	2	3	—	3	—	18
9-10 yrs.	11	3	2	1	3	—	20
10-11 yrs.	7	2	2	—	2	—	13
11-12 yrs.	5	—	1	—	—	—	6
12-13 yrs.	4	1	—	—	—	—	5
13-14 yrs.	2	—	—	—	—	—	2
14-15 yrs.	—	—	—	—	1	—	1
Total	113	27	29	12	35	4	220
	140			41			

Seven patients were alive with metastases, all more than four years after resection. Three of these seven patients presented seven to ten years after lobectomy with a pulmonary tumour, visible at bronchoscopy, in a bronchus on the side opposite to that on which lobectomy was undertaken; in each instance the histological features of the new tumour were similar to those of the original— all were squamous. If these patients had not had a previous lobectomy, the radiographic and bronchoscopic appearances related to the new contralateral tumour would be accepted as those of primary bronchial carcinoma rather than carcinoma which had presented in a bronchus as the consequence of bronchial erosion from mediastinal glands. These three tumours may, therefore, represent new tumours rather than metastases. All were irradiated; one patient was alive three years after irradiation and 11 years after lobectomy.

In Table XVI the histology of the tumours managed by lobectomy is related to survival time in 220 patients known to be alive and well without clinically or radiographically recognisable metastases at the present time. The longest to survive was submitted to lobectomy for adenocarcinoma 15 years ago, at a time when lobectomy was rarely undertaken for bronchial carcinoma, or for a peripheral pulmonary lesion without pre-operative histological confirmation of the diagnosis of carcinoma but which could reasonably only be called a carcinoma. Survival for 5 or 10 years after lobectomy for a squamous or undifferentiated tumour with glandular metastases is not uncommon. Of those who have survived lobectomy for more than six years, 15 are over 70 years of age at the present time, and a further five are over 80 years; lobectomy in these patients appears to have little detrimental effect on longevity.

Some of those at present alive more than two but less than five years after lobectomy will almost certainly die from metastases, as will some of those alive more than five years after lobectomy and apparently entirely well at the present time. Of 470 patients submitted to lobectomy for carcinoma, 220 (47 per cent) were alive more than two years after lobectomy, without clinical or radiographic evidence of metastases. Of 351 patients submitted to lobectomy more than five years ago 134 (38 per cent) were alive and well, without evidence of metastases.

MANAGEMENT BY SEGMENTAL RESECTION

Segmental resection was undertaken in 17 patients. At no time in the period under discussion was segmental resection regarded as an acceptable alternative to, say, lobectomy in the management of established bronchial carcinoma, and the circumstances in which segmental resection was undertaken in these 17 patients were unusual. In all, the tumour was peripheral in type and the appearances at bronchoscopy were normal. Presentation in five symptomless patients was with an abnormal chest radiograph made for routine purposes, and in one patient presentation was with the symptoms of hypertrophic pulmonary osteoarthropathy. The peripheral spherical pulmonary shadow in three patients measured 1 cm. in transverse diameter and in only two patients was the pulmonary opacity greater than 2 cm. in diameter. In 12 patients the tumour was squamous in type, in one undifferentiated, and in four patients the tumour was an adenocarcinoma. The reasons for management of bronchial carcinoma by segmental resection were (a) interpretation by palpation of the lesion in seven patients as tuberculous; (b) separation of the resected segment from neighbouring segments by an anatomically complete fissure in five patients in whom the lesion was recognised as most probably carcinoma, but in whom it was judged as effective to manage the tumour by segmental resection as by lobectomy; and (c) severe limitation of respiratory reserve in five patients, in whom thoracotomy was undertaken with a view to doing the most limited resection possible to establish a diagnosis of carcinoma. Management of bronchial carcinoma by segmental resection in this small group of patients was followed by long survival in a proportion of patients not noticeably different from that which follows resection of greater extent for tumours of the same relatively small size. Since in none of the patients managed by segmental resection were hilar glands resected for histological examination and since none of the operative notes contains specific comment on the presence or absence of such glands, it is not possible to relate survival to the absence of hilar glandular invasion, although this remains a reasonable assumption. The pattern of emergence of metastatic tumour or recurrence of tumour at the site of resection or in the mediastinum was also not noticeably different in those managed by segmental resection from those which follow resection of greater extent. Of the 17 patients five were alive more than five years after segmental resection, undertaken in three for squamous carcinoma and in two for adenocarcinoma.

39

THE HISTOLOGY OF BRONCHIAL CARCINOMA IN PATIENTS WHO PRESENTED WITHOUT SYMPTOMS AND WITH AN ABNORMAL ROUTINE CHEST RADIOGRAPH, MADE FOR UNRELATED PURPOSE

Of 4,000 patients with bronchial carcinoma 192 (17 women and 175 men) were investigated because they were found at mass radiography—made for an unrelated routine purpose—to have an abnormal chest radiograph. A further large number of patients came for investigation with an abnormal film from a mass radiography unit, but these patients had been referred for radiography, usually by a general practitioner, because of respiratory or other symptoms and are not included in the figure of 192. The pulmonary tumour in 128 patients was peripheral in type—that is, in only one-third was there a bronchoscopic abnormality. The histological features were those of squamous carcinoma in 107, of which 67 were peripheral tumours; in 45 the tumour was called undifferentiated ("oat cell" in three of these) and 22 of these were peripheral; in 15 the tumour was an adenocarcinoma, peripheral in all but one; and in four the tumour was an alveolar cell carcinoma, peripheral and an isolated, well-defined opacity in all; in 21 patients, all with peripheral shadows, a histological diagnosis was not achieved, but collateral evidence made the diagnosis of carcinoma the only tenable one.

Of the 15 patients with an adenocarcinoma one, in whom a cervical gland contained tumour, was not treated surgically; he died six months after irradiation. The others were managed surgically, 12 by lobectomy, one by pneumonectomy and one by segmental resection. Of those submitted to lobectomy four are alive—nine, seven, four and two years after resection respectively; one, a woman, returned seven years after lobectomy with a new ipsilateral shadow, management of which was by completion of pneumonectomy, and the tumour was now called an alveolar cell carcinoma, differing widely in histological appearance from the original lesion—she remains well; the other patients have all died from metastases.

Omitting the patient mentioned above whose second tumour was an alveolar cell carcinoma, there were four patients with alveolar cell tumours, of whom one, a non-smoking woman, is alive seven years after lobectomy, the second is alive seven years after pneumonectomy (in his case mediastinal glands were invaded), and two were alive, five and three years, respectively, after lobectomy.

The tumour in 45 patients was an undifferentiated carcinoma. In 10 of these management was other than surgical and all had died within a year of investigation. In one patient submitted to exploratory thoracotomy the tumour was found to be irresectable; in the remaining 34 a resection was undertaken—lobectomy in 16 and pneumonectomy in 18. Of those submitted to lobectomy five were alive, two of them seven years after operation, both these two having had mediastinal glandular metastases demonstrable at the time of operation. Three patients were alive after pneumonectomy, two of them eight years after operation.

Of the 107 patients with squamous tumours 89 were managed surgically—42 by lobectomy, 36 by pneumonectomy, four by segmental resection, and in seven the tumour was irresectable. Of those managed only by lobectomy 19 are alive and well—three for five years after operation, three for seven years, four for eight years, three for nine years, one for eleven years and one for fourteen years after operation, and four for less than five years but for more than two years after operation. Five of the primary tumours in these 19 patients were less than 4 cm. in diameter and the smallest was 1 cm. in diameter. In three, including two who are now long survivors, mediastinal glands were invaded. Segmental resection in four patients has been followed by survival for eight years in two, and pneumonectomy for squamous carcinoma in 36 patients has been followed by long survival in seven, one of whom, alive eight years after operation, had mediastinal glandular metastases.

From this brief analysis of 192 patients referred because of an abnormal mass miniature or other chest radiograph, some facts emerge. There is no significant difference in the age distribution of this group of patients from that of the series as a whole. The number of peripheral tumours is significantly higher and the number of undifferentiated tumours significantly lower than in the series as a whole; peripheral squamous tumours, often small in size, and adenocarcinomata were relatively common. The number of patients submitted to thoracotomy is also significantly higher—only 50 (26 per cent), of whom 10 declined thoracotomy, were not managed surgically. Resection was frustrated in eight patients and complete in 144, of whom seven died as a direct consequence of thoracotomy—an operative mortality and a rate of irresectability each of about 5 per cent—figures significantly lower than in the series as a whole. Long survival amongst those who withstood resection was 40 per cent —again higher than in the series as a whole.

SMOKING HABITS IN RELATION TO HISTOLOGY

Of the 4,000 patients in this series 73 per cent are known to have smoked cigarettes. The records are not sufficiently precise to be able to classify this group into heavy, moderate and light smokers. Included as cigarette smokers are those who smoked a pipe or cigars in addition to cigarettes; also included are 28 patients who had stopped smoking 10 to 20 years before the clinical evidence of bronchial carcinoma was recognised, and 43 men who had stopped smoking 3 to 10 years before the diagnosis of bronchial carcinoma was made. Of the 4,000 patients, 3 per cent smoked only a pipe, and 4 per cent—62 women and 99 men—claimed never to have smoked. Amongst the women in the series (403 patients), therefore, 15 per cent claimed never to have smoked. The 4 per cent accepted as non-smokers includes only those regarding whose smoking habits there is no reasonable doubt. The tumour in the 161 non-smokers was squamous in 58, undifferentiated in 79, an adenocarcinoma in 13 and, in 11, of unknown histological type.

The smoking habits of 20 per cent of the 4,000 patients are not recorded.

41

ADENOCARCINOMA

Of 4,000 patients with a bronchial carcinoma, 202 were shown to have an adenocarcinoma and in 10 more a tumour of mixed histology was shown to include an adenocarcinoma. Amongst those patients shown to have an adenocarcinoma 13 did not smoke; 15 presented without respiratory symptoms and because of an abnormality found on routine chest radiography made for unrelated purpose; 11 presented with the symptoms and signs of hypertrophic pulmonary osteoarthropathy. Of the 212 patients with an adenocarcinoma 39 were women. The incidence of adenocarcinoma in the series as a whole is 5·3 per cent. Of the 4,000 patients 403 were women, an incidence of bronchial carcinoma amongst women in the series of 10 per cent. The incidence of adenocarcinoma amongst women was 19 per cent—a significantly higher incidence of adenocarcinoma in women. Of 212 patients with adenocarcinoma management by pulmonary resection was completed in 110 (pneumonectomy in 35, of whom four were women, lobectomy in 71, of whom 15 were women, and segmental resection in four, all of whom were men), and in a further 15 patients an attempt at resection was abandoned after exploratory thoracotomy —two of these were women. Of 212 patients, therefore, 125, of whom 21 were women, were regarded after preliminary investigation as suitable for management by exploratory thoracotomy, and only 87 were regarded as unsuitable for this form of management—on the grounds of cervical glandular metastases in 42 (5 women), of cerebral metastases in nine (three women), on the grounds of pleural metastases with effusion in seven (four women), of pulmono-pulmonary metastases in three (one woman), and on the grounds of other metastases or other evidences of unsuitability for surgical management in 26, of whom five were women.

In comparison with the series as a whole it can, therefore, be said that pulmonary adenocarcinoma presented disproportionately often with hypertrophic pulmonary osteoarthropathy; was symptomless and was found by chance at routine radiography for an unrelated purpose in a disproportionately large number of patients; was significantly more common amongst women but probably not significantly more common amongst non-smokers; was, after routine pre-operative investigation, considered significantly more commonly to be suitable for surgical management, and in particular management by lobectomy, in comparison with other histological types; and despite the high incidence of resectability, was associated with death from metastases, and in particular from cerebral metastases, within the first two years of operation, disconcertingly frequently. Where adenocarcinoma had disseminated, clinical evidence of dissemination to cervical glands and thoracoscopic evidence of dissemination to the pleura, particularly amongst women, was disproportionately frequent. On the whole haematogenous dissemination from adenocarcinoma is more common than from other histological types of bronchial carcinoma, and more common than lymphatic dissemination.

ALVEOLAR CELL CARCINOMA

Of a small number of patients (17) with alveolar cell carcinoma 12 were suitable for surgical management—pneumonectomy in five and lobectomy in seven. Two of the 12 surgically managed were women. In two other patients, not included in the total of 12, alveolar cell carcinoma was demonstrated as part of mixed histology—one patient managed by pneumonectomy had an alveolar cell carcinoma the glandular metastases from which showed the features of adenocarcinoma and one patient managed by lobectomy had a primary tumour the bronchoscopic biopsy from which showed the features of squamous carcinoma, the operative specimen of which showed the features of adenocarcinoma, and glandular metastases from which showed the features of alveolar cell carcinoma. Four of the five patients with alveolar cell carcinoma who were managed by pneumonectomy and one of those managed by lobectomy, had mediastinal glandular metastases. All the alveolar cell carcinomas managed surgically were peripheral in type except where alveolar cell carcinoma was part of a mixed tumour. Of those managed by pneumonectomy, one died from a cause not related to metastases, one died from metastases within six months of operation and three, all with invaded mediastinal glands, were alive and well at the time of making this survey, in the second, third and seventh years, respectively, after pneumonectomy. Of those managed by lobectomy, one died as a direct consequence of operation and one died from metastases within a year of operation. A third was alive at the time of this survey, but with metastases, and four were well four, five, seven and eight years respectively, after lobectomy, the longest survivor having had mediastinal glandular metastases at the time of operation.

Four patients with peripheral alveolar cell tumours presented without symptoms and with an abnormal radiograph made for an unrelated purpose; a fifth patient, previously submitted to lobectomy for adenocarcinoma, returned with a new pulmonary opacity on the same side as the previous operation; management was by completion of pneumonectomy and the new or recurrent tumour was called an alveolar cell carcinoma.

Five patients with alveolar cell tumours were unsuitable for surgical management when first they were seen; one of these patients presented with bilateral spontaneous pneumothorax, under tension on one side. Death in these five patients was within very few weeks of first presentation to hospital and was related directly to advance of the tumour. From this small series of patients with alveolar cell carcinoma, the operability rate and the incidence of long survival are surprisingly high, and the behaviour of the tumour does not seem to justify its malignant reputation.

THE HISTOLOGY OF BRONCHIAL CARCINOMA IN PATIENTS UNSUITABLE FOR SURGICAL MANAGEMENT

In Table XVII the histology of tumours in patients unsuitable for surgical management is listed.

TABLE XVII

Histology of Bronchial Carcinoma in Patients Unsuitable for Surgical Management

	Sq.	U.	Ad.	Alv.	Mixed	Un-known	Total
Cervical glandular metastases	87	216	42	—		—	345
Lymphangitis carcinomatosa	17	7	—	—		—	24
Cerebral metastases	45	63	9	—		16	133
Osseous metastases	26	39	—	—		22	87
Hepatic metastases	23	40	—	—		3	66
Pulmono-pulmonary metastases	23	8	3	—		8	42
Superior vena caval obstruction	53	109	1	—		20	183
Mediastinal invasion (oesophageal displacement, phrenic paresis or both)	70	129	1	1		21	222
Mediastinal invasion (left recurrent laryngeal nerve palsy)	49	26	2	—		55	132
Metastases in skin, muscle, scars etc.	33	24	3	2		—	62
Endoscopic contra-indication	71	104	4	—		—	179
Impaired respiratory function	61	23	—	—		31	115
Age and frailty	46	22	—	—		6	74
Cardiac disease	13	13	1	—		—	27
Concomitant pulmonary dis. (asthma, tuberculosis, bronchiectasis etc.)	30	9	—	—		—	39
Declined treatment or died during investigation	58	64	2	2		25	151
Chest wall invasion including Pancoast's tumour	41	20	—	—		25	86
Pleural metastases	41	34	7	—		—	82
Multiple evidence of spread not included elsewhere	60	106	2	—		—	168
	847	1056	77	5	—	232	2217
Surgically managed	1054	536	125	12	56	—	1783
	1901	1592	202	17	56	232	4000

An ipsilateral cervical glandular metastasis was the only contra-indication to surgical management in 190 patients and in over 60 per cent of these tumours were undifferentiated. The cervical glandular metastasis was one of several contra-indications to surgical management in 234 patients and in one-third of these the tumour was undifferentiated. In 77 patients contra-lateral cervical glandular metastases were found—in 46 of these the tumour was undifferentiated, in 24 squamous, and in seven an adenocarcinoma. In 44 patients the pulmonary primary was on the left and the cervical gland on the right, and in 33 patients the pulmonary primary was on the right and the cervical gland on the left. In 78 patients cervical glandular metastases were bilateral and in 50 of these the tumour was undifferentiated, in 25 squamous and in three an adenocarcinoma. Adenocarcinoma presented with cervical glandular metastases in 42 patients, five of whom were women—that is, 20 per cent of all patients with adenocarcinoma presented with cervical glandular metastases, which is a percentage disproportionately high when compared with the series as a whole. Of those patients with contra-lateral cervical glandular metastases there was other evidence of wide-spread dissemination of tumour in 54 and bilateral cervical glandular metastases was the only evidence of tumour dissemination in only five of 78 patients.

The radiographic appearances interpreted as those of lymphangitis carcinomatosa were seen in 24 patients with bronchial carcinoma; in seven of these the radiographic appearances were the only evidence of dissemination of tumour; in 17 the tumour was a squamous carcinoma and in the remainder an undifferentiated carcinoma.

Of 133 patients who presented with cerebral metastases a histological diagnosis was ultimately achieved in all but 16. The tumour was called undifferentiated in 63, squamous in 45 and in 9 the tumour was an adenocarcinoma.

Of 87 patients who presented with osseous metastases histological confirmation of the diagnosis of bronchial carcinoma was achieved in all but 22. In 26 the tumour was squamous and in 39 undifferentiated. Osseous metastases were found in 48 other patients who had evidence of extra-pulmonary dissemination of tumour in addition to osseous metastases. In only one patient, with osseous and cervical glandular metastases, is the primary pulmonary tumour known to have been an adenocarcinoma.

Hepatic metastases were found as the only contra-indication to surgical management in 66 patients with bronchial carcinoma. Histological confirmation of the diagnosis was achieved in 63 of the 66 patients; in 40 the tumour was called undifferentiated and in 23 squamous.

Forty-two patients were found, when first they presented for investigation, to have radiographic evidence of pulmono-pulmonary metastases as the only evidence of spread of tumour. The histological pattern of the tumour is known in 34 of the 42 patients. Squamous tumours in 15 patients, undifferentiated tumours in four and adenocarcinomata in three patients were visible at bronchoscopy; cervical lymph glandular metastases from four peripheral squamous and two undifferentiated tumours developed later and were proven histologically; two patients who were submitted to pulmonary biopsy were shown to have squamous tumours; in four patients in whom the histological features of the tumour were unknown before death, necropsy allowed of the making of the diagnosis of squamous carcinoma in two and undifferentiated carcinoma in the other two. Nearly three in every four of the tumours the histology of which is known were shown, therefore, to be squamous in type.

Of 4,000 patients with bronchial carcinoma 183 had, at the time of first presentation, the clinical features of obstruction of the superior vena cava. Histological confirmation of the diagnosis of bronchial carcinoma was obtained in 163 of 183 patients; in 109 the tumour was undifferentiated, in 53 squamous and in only one an adenocarcinoma. The proportion of undifferentiated to squamous tumours is unusually high, when compared with the series as a whole.

In 138 patients displacement of the barium-filled oesophagus, recognised at fluoroscopy and recorded radiographically, was the only evidence of tumour extension beyond the lung. In 39 patients the tumour was a squamous carcinoma, in 80 an undifferentiated carcinoma; in one the tumour was an adenocarcinoma and in one other an alveolar cell carcinoma; in 17 the tumour was peripheral in type, without bronchoscopic abnormality, and in these histological confirmation of the diagnosis was not achieved at the time of irradiation; in seven of the 17 necropsy, four to 17 months after irradiation, supplied the histological diagnosis—of undifferentiated carcinoma in four and of squamous carcinoma in three.

In 65 patients with bronchial carcinoma phrenic paresis was the only evidence of extension of tumour beyond the lung. In 35 patients the tumour was called undifferentiated, and in 21 squamous: in nine a histological diagnosis was not achieved.

Nineteen patients, all men, were shown to have both oesophageal displacement and interruption of the phrenic nerve as the only evidence of extension of tumour outwith the lung. In 17 the tumour was central, and of these the tumour was squamous in 7 and undifferentiated in 10.

In 132 patients, bronchial carcinoma was associated with interruption of the left recurrent laryngeal nerve as the only evidence of extra-pulmonary extension of tumour. The tumour was visible at bronchoscopy in only 47, in 26 of whom the histological features were those of squamous carcinoma, in 19 of an undifferentiated tumour and in two of an adenocarcinoma. Ultimate histological proof of the diagnosis was obtained in a further 30 patients, in 23 of whom the tumour was squamous. Where histological proof of the diagnosis of bronchial carcinoma was achieved in relation to left recurrent laryngeal nerve palsy, the tumour was, therefore, often squamous and slow growing, since survival from the onset of hoarseness of voice was often surprisingly long.

Cutaneous or subcutaneous metastases were found in 38 patients in whom this was the only evidence of dissemination of bronchial carcinoma, and in 19 others in conjunction with additional clinical evidence of spread. Metastases in muscle were encountered in eight patients and in scars in three patients. Two men presented with purpura and splenomegaly and had tumour in bone marrow, and an abdominal mass other than hepatic in nine patients was established as the consequence of metastases of bronchial carcinoma— squamous in four and undifferentiated in five. Unusual sites of metastases were the scalp, the tongue, a tonsil, the hard palate, the lower alveolus, a thumb and a second toe.

Of 4,000 patients with bronchial carcinoma 179 were not managed surgically because of an endoscopic contra-indication. In four the tumour was an adenocarcinoma, in 71 squamous and in 104 undifferentiated. In 132 of the 179 patients the tumour was right-sided—a disproportionate emphasis on the right in comparison with the series as a whole. In three of these patients the tumour was in the trachea and the accompanying radiograph was normal.

Respiratory function in 115 patients (112 men) with pulmonary carcinoma was so poor that a thoracotomy was precluded. In 88 histological confirmation of the diagnosis was achieved—the tumour was squamous in 61, undifferentiated in 23 and of unspecified cell type, the cells being recognised in sputa in eight. In none was the diagnosis of adenocarcinoma made. Many patients with peripheral tumours died before the tumour had reached a large size and without clinical evidence of metastases and it is suggested that these patients died with rather than from, bronchial carcinoma.

Bronchial carcinoma in 14 patients was not managed surgically because in each it was associated with extensive active pulmonary tuberculosis. The tumour in nine of the 14 patients in this group was squamous and in five undifferentiated. One of these patients was a boy of 19 years, in whom the pulmonary tumour was undifferentiated.

Bronchial carcinoma in six patients with severe chronic asthma, squamous in all, was not treated in any way because of asthma. In eight patients extensive pneumoconiosis alone precluded thoracotomy—in all the tumour was squamous. Four men with squamous tumours were not managed surgically because of bullous emphysema. Known bronchiectasis in three patients precluded surgical management for squamous carcinoma in one and undifferentiated carcinoma in two. Advanced chronological age alone in 38 patients precluded surgical management; in 32 of these the histological diagnosis was established and in 22 the tumour was squamous and in 10 undifferentiated.

In 27 patients myocardial disease alone precluded surgical management. In 13 the tumour was a squamous carcinoma and in 13 an undifferentiated carcinoma; in one, in whom histological confirmation of the diagnosis of carcinoma was achieved only at necropsy, the tumour was an adenocarcinoma. In the case records of 36 patients, 24 with squamous tumours and 12 with undifferentiated tumours, frailty or " decrepitude " alone is recorded as having precluded surgical management.

An undifferentiated carcinoma was managed by radiotherapy in a man in a plaster jacket; a squamous carcinoma was managed by irradiation in a man with syringomyelia, and a squamous carcinoma was managed by irradiation in a man previously treated for oesophageal carcinoma and aortic aneurysm. One man with " oat cell " carcinoma was irradiated as part of an M.R.C. trial.

Of 80 patients who declined treatment, the tumour in 35 was squamous, in six undifferentiated and in 27 the histology was unknown. Seventy-four patients died during investigation, most from cardio-vascular disease or pulmonary infection, two from complications related to investigation.

In 49 patients with medial invasion of the chest wall the tumour was squamous in 27 and undifferentiated in 14. In 37 patients with Pancoast's syndrome the tumour was squamous in 14 and undifferentiated in six and unknown in the remainder.

In 82 patients pleural metastases were the only evidence of dissemination of bronchial carcinoma; 23 were women. In 41 the tumour was squamous, in 34 undifferentiated and in seven an adenocarcinoma. The number of women and the number of adenocarcinomata is, therefore, disproportionately high.

In 49 patients who presented with hypertrophic pulmonary osteoarthropathy the tumour was squamous in 25, undifferentiated in 13 and an adenocarcinoma in 11.

V

The Influence of Age on the Results of Management

SUMMARY

There is statistical evidence of an increasing incidence of bronchial carcinoma in those over 70 years and possibly of a diminishing incidence amongst those under 50 years.

Surgical management of bronchial carcinoma was associated with a higher early post-operative mortality amongst the aged. The operative mortality in those in the fifth decade, managed by pneumonectomy, was half that in those in the seventh decade; the operative mortality in the sixth decade was half that in the eighth decade; amongst those younger than 60 years the operative mortality was half that amongst those 60 years and over; the operative mortality in those 65 years and over was 20 per cent in comparison with an overall operative mortality of 12 per cent.

In those managed by lobectomy the operative mortality amongst those younger than 65 years was one-third of the operative mortality in those 65 years and older, and in those over 70 years was 22 per cent—three times the operative mortality for all patients managed by lobectomy.

Patients who presented with obstruction of the superior vena cava were more commonly women and of a younger age than would be anticipated from the overall age range.

Management by exploratory thoracotomy was precluded on the ground of diminished respiratory reserve in nearly 4 per cent of the whole series of 4,000 patients, and most of these patients were over 60 years of age. In 1 per cent of all patients advanced age alone precluded surgical management, and nearly all these patients were older than 75 years. Frailty precluded surgical management in a further 1 per cent, the age of all of whom was relatively advanced.

THE purpose of this chapter is to present the facts which relate to age and to assess the influence of age on the results of management of bronchial carcinoma in 4,000 consecutive patients.

The facts which relate to age and sex are graphically illustrated in Figures 4-7. Of 4,000 patients 403 (10 per cent) were women. The youngest patients were a girl of 16 and a boy and a girl of 19; the oldest was a man of 91 years. In this series bronchial carcinoma was most common in the sixth and seventh decades; 22 per cent of women and 15 per cent of men were younger than 50 years, and 11 per cent of women and 10 per cent of men were 70 years or older (Fig. 4). The first 2,000 patients were investigated between the beginning

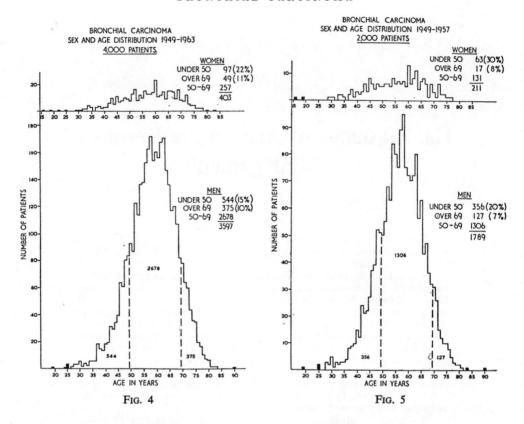

FIG. 4

FIG. 5

of 1949 and the beginning of 1957. In this group of 2,000 patients (Fig. 5) 30 per cent of women and 20 per cent of men were younger than 50 years of age, and only 8 per cent of women and 7 per cent of men were 70 years or older. The second group of 2,000 patients (Fig. 6) was investigated between February 1957 and November 1963. In this second group 17 per cent of women and 10 per cent of men were younger than 50 years at the time of investigation, and 16 per cent of women and 14 per cent of men were 70 years or older. In the second half of the series, therefore, the incidence of bronchial carcinoma in men and women of 70 years and older had doubled—an observation probably explicable on the ground of an ageing population. But in the second half of the series the incidence of the disease in those younger than 50 years had diminished—by half amongst the men and by a little less than half amongst the women. It has been observed (Fletcher, 1966, personal communication) that the mortality of bronchial carcinoma in younger people is diminishing; an adequate explanation for this observed fact cannot yet be offered. It is an interesting conjecture that an immunity to the disease is developing. In Figure 7, Figures 5 and 6 are superimposed, making clear the shift of the disease to the older age groups.

50

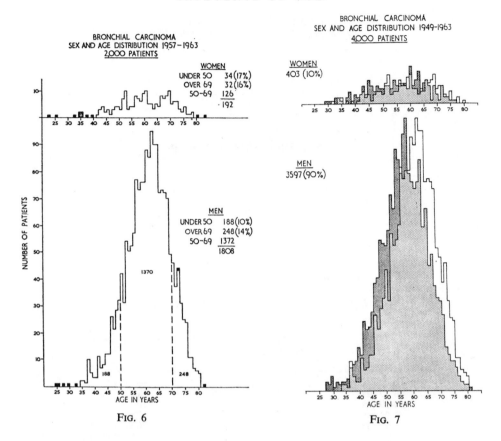

FIG. 6

FIG. 7

INFLUENCE OF AGE ON THE RESULTS OF SURGICAL MANAGEMENT

Exploration at Thoracotomy without Resection. Thoracotomy with a view to resection of pulmonary carcinoma was undertaken in 319 patients (8 per cent) in whom the tumour was found to be either technically irresectable or to be associated with evidence of dissemination which made pulmonary resection pointless. The age incidence in this group is shown in Figure 8. Death could be related to operation in 20 patients, all of them men. Exploration only, without pulmonary resection, is therefore, in this series, associated with an operative mortality of 6 per cent. Of patients over 60 years, 8 per cent died; of those younger than 60 years, 5 per cent died; of those 55 years of age or younger only 3 per cent died.

Management by Pneumonectomy. Bronchial carcinoma in 977 patients (24 per cent) was managed by pneumonectomy. The relation between the histological type of the tumour and the age of the patients has been shown in Figure 2. Between the ages of 45 and 70, for any half decade, squamous tumours occurred with a frequency a little less than three times that of undiffer-

51

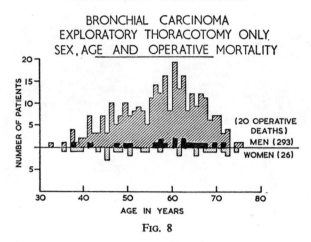

BRONCHIAL CARCINOMA
EXPLORATORY THORACOTOMY ONLY
SEX, AGE AND OPERATIVE MORTALITY

(20 OPERATIVE DEATHS)
MEN (293)
WOMEN (26)

Fig. 8

TABLE XVIII

Pneumonectomy (906 Men)

Operative Mortality in Relation to Age

Age	Number of operations	Number of deaths	Percentage operative mortality
Under 40 yrs.	26	—	—
40-49 yrs.	130	10	8%
50-59 yrs.	396	40	10%
60-69 yrs.	307	54	17%
70-79 yrs,	47	9	20%
Total	906	113	12%
Under 60 yrs.	552	50	9%
60 yrs. & over	354	63	18%
65 yrs. & over	175	35	20%

entiated tumours; under the age of 40 years squamous tumours, amongst a small total number of patients, were less common than undifferentiated tumours; over the age of 70 years, again amongst only a small total number of patients, five in every six tumours were squamous.

Age at the time of pneumonectomy is shown in Figure 9. Of the 977 patients managed by pneumonectomy 71 (7 per cent) were women. The graphic pattern of age, as shown in Figure 9 is not significantly different from that which shows the age distribution of the series as a whole (Figs. 4-7) but in comparison with that which shows the age of those found suitable for management by lobectomy (Fig. 10) relatively fewer over the age of 70 years were suitable for management by pneumonectomy than were suitable for management by lobectomy. Eight women and 113 men died as a direct consequence of pneumonectomy for bronchial carcinoma—an overall operative mortality

PNEUMONECTOMY FOR BRONCHIAL CARCINOMA
SEX, AGE AND OPERATIVE MORTALITY

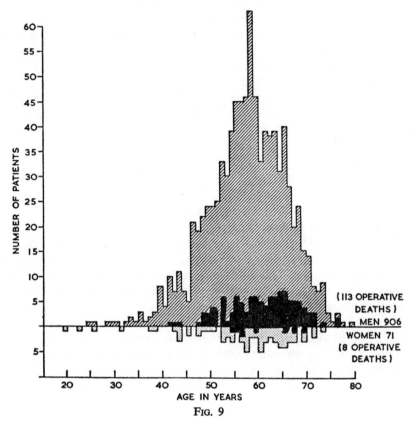

FIG. 9

LOBECTOMY FOR BRONCHIAL CARCINOMA
SEX, AGE AND OPERATIVE MORTALITY

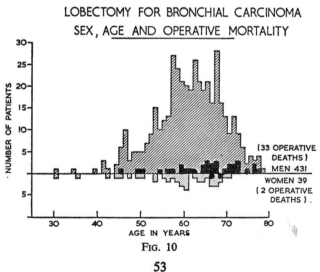

FIG. 10

53

of 12 per cent, an operative mortality amongst men of 12 per cent and amongst women of 10 per cent. Operative mortality amongst men in relation to age is shown in Table XVIII and it is clear that the operative mortality rate increased with age. The operative mortality in the fifth decade was half that in the seventh decade; the operative mortality in the sixth decade was half that in the eighth decade; the operative mortality amongst those younger than 60 years was half that amongst those 60 years and over; the operative mortality in those 65 years and over was 20 per cent.

The three common causes of death in the post-operative period after pneumonectomy were respiratory infection, coronary thrombosis and pulmonary embolism. Only 3 of 22 patients who died from coronary thrombosis after pneumonectomy were younger than 50 years. The two oldest were 70 and 71 years respectively.

Management by Lobectomy. Bronchial carcinoma in 470 (12 per cent) was managed by lobectomy—in 91 of these by the resection of two lobes and in 61 by lobectomy with resection of a length of stem bronchus. Only 18 per cent of tumours managed by lobectomy were undifferentiated; 65 per cent were squamous and 15 per cent were adenocarcinomata. Age at the time of lobectomy is shown in Figure 10. Of the 470 patients managed in this way 39 (8 per cent) were women. The graphic pattern of age as shown in Figure 10 is not significantly different from that which shows the age distribution in the series as a whole (Figs. 4-7) but in comparison with Figure 9 which illustrates the age distribution of patients managed by pneumonectomy, more patients over the age of 70 years were suitable for management of bronchial carcinoma by lobectomy than by pneumonectomy. Two women and 33 men died as a direct consequence of operation—an operative mortality of 7 per cent. Operative mortality in relation to age is shown in Table XIX and it is clear that the operative mortality increased with age. The operative mortality in

TABLE XIX

Lobectomy (Men)

Operative Mortality in Relation to Age

Age	Number of operations	Number of deaths	Percentage operative mortality
30-39 yrs.	3	—	—
40-49 yrs.	35	—	—
50-59 yrs.	143	7	4%
60-69 yrs.	199	15	7%
70-78 yrs.	51	11	22%
Total	431	33	8%
Over 65 yrs.	145	20	14%
Under 65 yrs.	286	13	4·5%

those younger than 65 years was 4·5 per cent and in those 65 years or older was 14 per cent, while in those 70 years or over the operative mortality was 22 per cent.

AGE IN THOSE WITH DISSEMINATED TUMOUR

Management in 1,834 (45·9 per cent) patients was other than surgical because of clinical, radiographic, fluoroscopic, bronchoscopic or thoracoscopic evidence of metastases or extra-pulmonary extension of tumour. The range of age in this group was unremarkable and not significantly different from that in the group managed by resection, except in those who presented with obstruction of the superior vena cava, amongst whom there was a disproportionately large number of women and a disproportionately large number (58 per cent) younger than 60 years, notwithstanding a deliberate attempt at limiting the number of patients in this group in order to avoid the inclusion of any patient who might have a lymphoma

AGE IN THOSE MANAGED OTHER THAN BY OPERATION FOR REASONS OTHER THAN METASTATIC

Respiratory function in 115 (2·9 per cent) of 4,000 patients was so poor that thoracotomy was precluded on this ground alone, there being no other contra-indication to surgical management. Of the 115 patients 112 were men of whom 23 per cent were older than 69 years (in comparison with 10 per cent in the series as a whole) and 75 per cent were older than 59 years (in comparison with 48 per cent of all men in the series). Impairment of respiratory reserve of a degree which precluded surgical management was therefore commonly related to advanced age—which is precisely what could reasonably be anticipated.

In 38 patients age was accepted as the only contra-indication to surgical management of bronchial carcinoma. Of the 38 patients 35 were men. Chronological age alone is difficult to define as a bar to surgical management—if 80 is too old, is 79 also too old? The relation between age and post-operative mortality amongst patients in whom bronchial carcinoma was managed by resection has already been presented in detail and there is no doubt that a higher proportion of older patients die in convalescence from pulmonary resection. Of the 38 patients regarded as too old for surgical management, 30 were 75 years or older and four were 80 years old. Most were not only chronologically but also physiologically old—two patients of 80 years were, however, in remarkably good physiological condition. All these patients had died five months to two and a half years from the time of investigation, and it is the impression that some at least died with rather than from bronchial carcinoma.

In the case records of 36 patients, all with histologically established bronchial carcinoma and without clinical, radiographic, fluoroscopic or bronchoscopic evidence of dissemination of tumour, the statement was made that, although measurement of respiratory function did not preclude management

55

of bronchial carcinoma by resection, " frailty " (or in some instances " decrepitude ") was such that, on general grounds, these patients were all regarded as unsuitable for surgical management—and indeed in some instances for treatment of any sort. The youngest patient in this group of 36 was 55 years; most were older than 65 years and the three oldest were 71 years of age. These patients were all discharged from hospital and died at home within six months of investigation. In none did the opportunity again arise for examination and in none was a post mortem examination undertaken, so that it is not possible to relate frailty in these patients to cryptic metastases or other disease of a degenerative nature. But there is no doubt that where frailty is recorded as a contra-indication to surgical management, this is usually a concomitant of relatively advanced age.

VI

Results of Surgical Management

SUMMARY

Exploratory thoracotomy was undertaken in 1,783 patients (44 per cent of the series): in 1,464 (36·6 per cent) pulmonary resection was completed and in 319 (8 per cent) resection was frustrated.

Exploration without pulmonary resection carried a mortality of 6 per cent and in the group of patients only explored the incidence of undifferentiated: squamous tumours was 9 : 10. Most who survived operation were managed by palliative irradiation; 71 per cent had died within a year of operation.

In 977 patients (24 per cent) the resection undertaken was pneumonectomy, the operative mortality for which was 12 per cent. The operative mortality rate increased with age, and was nearly twice as high for right as for left pneumonectomy. Two in every three tumours managed by pneumonectomy were central in type, and 60 per cent were squamous. Mediastinal glands were invaded in 41 per cent. Respiratory infection, coronary thrombosis and pulmonary embolism were the common causes of death in early convalescence, and one in every three patients who died from metastases in the first two years after pneumonectomy died with cerebral metastases. Of those submitted to pneumonectomy more than five years before completion of this analysis, 20 per cent were alive.

In 470 patients (12 per cent) the resection undertaken was lobectomy, the operative mortality for which was 7 per cent. The operative mortality rate increased with age, and was highest for right upper lobectomy. Where a single lobe was resected, five in every six tumours were peripheral in type, and 65 per cent of tumours managed by lobectomy were squamous. Of those submitted to lobectomy more than five years ago, 38 per cent. were alive.

Segmental resection was undertaken on 17 patients, five of whom were long survivors.

BRONCHIAL carcinoma in those patients in whom dissemination of tumour beyond a lung had not been demonstrated, who were, on general grounds suitable for pulmonary resection, and who accepted surgical management, were submitted to thoracotomy with a view to pulmonary resection. Management was by radiotherapy in most patients with metastases or who would not submit to an operation. Management has been outlined in Table III. Of 4,000 patients 44·6 per cent (1,783) were submitted to exploratory thoracotomy and some form of pulmonary resection was completed in 1,464 patients (36·6 per cent). Surgical management was precluded in 1,834 patients (45·9 per cent) because of clinical, radiographic, fluoroscopic or bronchoscopic evidence of dissemination of tumour, and in 383 (9·5 per cent) because of evidence of unsuitability for surgical management other than metastases, or because they declined operation. Management of bronchial carcinoma in relation to invasion of the chest wall, pleural effusion and empyema thoracis is separately discussed.

I. EXPLORATION AT THORACOTOMY WITHOUT RESECTION

Thoracotomy with a view to resection of pulmonary carcinoma was undertaken in 319 patients (8 per cent) in whom the tumour was found either to be technically irresectable or to be associated with evidence of dissemination of tumour which made pulmonary resection pointless. Of the 319 patients 26 were women and 293 were men, a male : female ratio of 11 : 1. The age incidence in this group has been shown in Figure 8. Death could be related more or less directly to operation in 20 patients, all of them men. Exploration only, without pulmonary resection, is therefore in this series associated with an operative mortality of 6 per cent. Post-operative death in this group was related to age—death in the post-operative period was a little more common in patients over 60, amongst whom 8 per cent of the patients died, than in those younger than 60, amongst whom 5 per cent of patients died; of those 55 years of age or younger, only 3 per cent died in the post-operative period.

The tumour was on the right in 165 patients and on the left in 154. In 197 patients histological confirmation of the diagnosis of bronchial carcinoma had been obtained before thoracotomy by a biopsy made at bronchoscopy—these patients had central tumours. The bronchoscopic appearances in 122 patients with tumours of peripheral type were normal. In 163 patients the tumour was squamous, and in 139 undifferentiated (in 28 of these called " oat-cell "). In 15 patients the tumour was an adenocarcinoma; in two patients with central tumours the tumour was typed histologically as squamous on the ground of the bronchoscopic biopsy and as an adenocarcinoma in one and an oat-cell carcinoma in the other on biopsy at operation. The ratio of undifferentiated to squamous carcinoma in this group of 319 patients is nearly 9 : 10—a disproportionately high incidence of undifferentiated tumours as compared with the series as a whole.

Death during convalescence was the consequence of pulmonary embolism in four patients; of pulmonary infection and respiratory insufficiency, the latter the consequence of pulmonary infection and thoracotomy, in seven patients; and of pulmonary and pleural infection together in one. Death in convalescence was a consequence of coronary thrombosis in two patients in both of whom there was a history of coronary thrombosis before operation and one of whom developed atrial fibrillation early in convalescence; of massive haemoptysis within four weeks of thoracotomy in two patients; of congestive cardiac failure in two patients; of renal shutdown in one; and in the last of acute obstruction of the superior vena cava by thrombus on the second post-operative day, the vena cava having been damaged during the attempt at mobilisation of the right pulmonary hilum.

Resection was not undertaken because it was technically impossible safely to control the hilar structures in 256 patients (80 per cent). Because of the possibility of controlling pulmonary veins intra-pericardially at atrial level, with the sacrifice of more or less of the atrium, proximal involvement of pulmonary artery or bronchus more often precluded resection than did proximal involvement of pulmonary veins. Invasion of prohibitive magnitude of superior vena cava or aorta, invasion of the chest wall in relation to vertebrae, or tumour so extensive that the mediastinum or heart was widely invaded and there were several individual reasons for not being able to complete resection, are all recorded in operative notes.

Resection was technically possible in 63 patients (20 per cent) but was not undertaken because it was regarded as pointless or dangerous. Reasons for regarding resection as pointless were: diffuse pleural metastases (27 patients); hepatic metastases appreciated by palpation of the liver through the diaphragm at thoracotomy (nine patients); massive glandular spread in relation to a small primary tumour (18 patients); cardiac metastases (in the wall of the left ventricle in two patients); diffuse, small and very numerous pulmonary metastases recognised neither pre-operatively nor in retrospect on chest radiographs (two patients); a pulmonary tumour of such an extent that pneumonectomy was technically necessary in a patient whose respiratory reserve was so limited that lobectomy was judged the maximum permissible resection (five patients). The 63 patients in whom resection was technically possible but in whom the primary tumour was not resected had this in common—the primary tumour was either symptomless or associated with symptoms which could be related to metastases first recognised at operation and which could not be resected. It was commonplace to undertake pulmonary resection for carcinoma in the presence of spread—often extensive—found at thoracotomy in patients with symptoms, in order to palliate symptoms, especially haemoptysis—in fact it was the general rule until 1957 to complete a pulmonary resection wherever this was technically possible, and this attitude was deliberately abandoned only when it could be shown from careful assessment of the subsequent course that a small and symptomless primary tumour found at thoracotomy to be related to unsuspected metastases did not grow and become the source of symptoms before death related to metastases ensued. Four patients in this group of 63 did not smoke.

Of the 299 patients in whom bronchial carcinoma was found unsuitable for management by resection at exploratory thoracotomy and who survived the period of immediate convalescence, 223 were subsequently managed by palliative irradiation, treatment in these beginning within two to three weeks of thoracotomy; 39 other patients were irradiated at a later stage after thoracotomy because of the emergence of symptoms, in most bone pain, which it was judged would respond to irradiation; five were given cytotoxic drugs intravenously during convalescence; and in eight cytotoxic drugs were instilled into the pleural space in an attempt to retard the growth of pleural metastases.

None of the 299 patients who survived early convalescence from thoracotomy was alive three years later. Forty-seven patients died within three months of thoracotomy—from massive haemoptysis during irradiation; acutely, as if from coronary thrombosis or similar cardiovascular catastrophe, but without evidence by necropsy of a cause of death; and by rapid decline as if from rapidly growing tumour—and in this group is included all those given cytotoxic drugs. A further 72 patients died within six months of thoracotomy, and a further 84 within a year of operation—that is, within 12 months of thoracotomy 213 (71 per cent) of patients in whom bronchial carcinoma had been found unsuitable for management by resection had died. Five patients died two to two and a half years after thoracotomy, and the rest died during the second year after exploration. All but three of those who lived for longer than a year had been irradiated during the first three months after thoracotomy.

Thoracotomy was undertaken in the knowledge that displacement of the barium-filled oesophagus had been demonstrated at fluoroscopy in a group of 30 patients, and in 23 of these the tumour was technically irresectable. Thoracotomy was undertaken in the knowledge that paradoxical movement of the ipsilateral diaphragmatic dome had been demonstrated in 17 patients and in five of these the tumour was irresectable. The circumstances in which these contra-indications to thoracotomy were ignored are discussed elsewhere in this analysis (pp. 109 and 110).

In seven patients in whom a left thoracotomy had been made for a tumour which was found to be irresectable, hoarseness of voice was recognised early in convalescence, and it is presumed that the left recurrent laryngeal nerve had been damaged during exploration of the pulmonary hilum. These seven patients had all of them a tumour which extended to occupy the concavity of the aortic arch—a common finding in patients with irresectable left pulmonary carcinoma. None of the standard forms of investigation allows of the pre-operative recognition of left pulmonary carcinoma inoperable because of proximal extension to occupy the concavity of the aortic arch or to involve the pulmonary artery medial to the ligamentum arteriosum, and limited experience with pneumomediastinography makes it unlikely that this will serve the purpose of allowing of unequivocal recognition of this degree of proximal extension of tumour.

II. MANAGEMENT BY PNEUMONECTOMY

Bronchial carcinoma in 977 patients (24 per cent) was managed by pneumonectomy—on the right in 462, and on the left in 515. The anatomical distribution of the tumours is shown in Table XX. In 290 patients the tumours were peripheral in type and in these the appearances at bronchoscopy were

TABLE XX

Pneumonectomy (977 Patients)

Anatomical Distribution of Tumours

(I) *Peripheral Tumours*

Right		Left		Total
Upper lobe	76	Upper lobe	117	193
Middle lobe	10			10
Lower lobe	27	Lower lobe	32	59
" Hilar "	7	" Hilar "	21	28
	120		170	290

(II) *Central Tumours*

Right		Left		Total
Upper lobe bronchus	140	Upper lobe bronchus	153	293
Main bronchus	12	Main bronchus	30	42
Intermediate bronchus	52			52
Middle lobe bronchus	14			14
Lower lobe bronchus	124	Lower lobe bronchus	162	286
	342		345	687

Right	462	Left	515	

normal. In this group the tumours were most commonly located in an upper lobe, more often in the left upper lobe. In 687 patients the tumour was central in type, and histological confirmation of the diagnosis of bronchial carcinoma was obtained in this group of patients by biopsy at bronchoscopy. Central tumours were as common in the upper as in the lower lobes, and on the right as on the left. Peripheral tumours were described as " hilar " when the radiographic shadow cast by the tumour was located at the pulmonary hilum on two radiographs made at right angles, and not certainly located in one lobe as opposed to another, and where, after resection, there remained doubt in which lobe to place the tumour. Central tumours apportioned to a lobe were visible in the appropriate lobar bronchus or in one of the segmental bronchi of that lobe, but might extend into the stem bronchus without importantly obstructing it. Tumours in the left main bronchus either obstructed it completely (in all instances more than 2 cm. distal to the main carina) or so nearly completely that a lobar origin could not be determined at bronchoscopy, and doubt remained regarding a precise lobar origin after scrutiny of the operative specimen. Tumours in the right main bronchus involved the lateral wall of the main bronchus proximal to the origin of the right upper bronchus, and in four instances extended on to the lateral wall of the trachea, but did not involve the medial wall or the main carina. Tumours in the intermediate bronchus partially or completely obstructed that length of stem bronchus distal to the lower lip of the right upper bronchus and proximal to the middle bronchus, and were usually associated with the radiographic appearances of shrinkage and airlessness of the middle and lower lobes.

The histological range in this group of 977 pneumonectomies has been discussed in Chapter IV. Squamous tumours were the most common (587); there were 311 undifferentiated tumours and only 35 adenocarcinomata; in five the tumour was alveolar, and in 39 patients the histological diagnosis from biopsy at bronchoscopy differed from the operative specimen or the mediastinal glands.

Mediastinal glands were invaded in 41 per cent of patients in whom pneumonectomy was undertaken—in 33 per cent with squamous tumours, in 55 per cent with undifferentiated tumours, in more than a third of the 35 patients with adenocarcinoma, in four of the five with alveolar cell tumours, and in nearly half of those in whom the cell-type was mixed. The incidence of lymph glandular metastases was higher for all histological types in patients submitted to pneumonectomy for peripheral tumours—46 per cent overall, 37 per cent with squamous tumours, and 58 per cent with undifferentiated tumours. The relationship between the histological type of the tumours and the age of the patients is shown in Figure 2. Between the ages of 45 and 70, for any half decade, squamous tumours occurred with a frequency a little less than three times that of undifferentiated tumours; under the age of 40 squamous tumours, amongst a small total number of patients, were less common than undifferentiated tumours; over the age of 70, again amongst only a small total number of patients, five in every six tumours were squamous.

Age at the time of pneumonectomy is shown in Figure 9. Of the 977 patients managed by pneumonectomy 71 (7 per cent) were women. The graphic pattern of age as shown in Figure 9 is not significantly different from that which shows the age distribution of the series as a whole (Figs. 4-7), but in comparison with that which shows the age of those found suitable for management by lobectomy (Fig. 10) relatively fewer over the age of 70 years are suitable for management by pneumonectomy than are suitable for management by lobectomy. Eight women and 113 men died as a direct consequence of pneumonectomy for bronchial carcinoma—an overall operative mortality of 12 per cent, an operative mortality amongst men of 12 per cent, and amongst women of 10 per cent. Operative mortality amongst men in relation to age is shown in Table XVIII, and it is clear that the operative mortality rate increased with age. The operative mortality in the fifth decade was half that in the seventh decade; the operative mortality in the sixth decade was half that in the eighth; the operative mortality amongst those younger than 60 years was half that amongst those 60 years and over; the operative mortality in those 65 years and over was 20 per cent.

Although left pneumonectomy was undertaken for bronchial carcinoma slightly more frequently than was right pneumonectomy, 77 patients died after right pneumonectomy and only 44 after left pneumonectomy. The tumour was squamous in 72 of those who died as a consequence of pneumonectomy, undifferentiated in 37, mixed in five and an adenocarcinoma in seven—an operative mortality highest in those with adenocarcinoma; the tumour was peripheral in 35 and central in 86 of those who died from pneumonectomy—an operative mortality relatively a little higher in those with peripheral tumours. There is little likelihood that the histological type of the tumour or the fact that a tumour was or was not visible at bronchoscopy had any significant bearing on operative mortality.

The three common causes of death in the post-operative period after pneumonectomy were respiratory infection, coronary thrombosis and pulmonary embolism. Of 121 patients who died after pneumonectomy, death in 47 was directly attributable to pulmonary infection. In 12 of these 47 respiratory reserve had been severely limited by pneumonectomy and pulmonary infection, albeit minor, so further diminished reserve that death ensued—an outcome less frequently seen in the last 10 years, during which recourse has been made to tracheostomy more frequently, and with less indication, and the range of antibiotics has become wider and more effective; in seven of the 47 empyema and broncho-pleural fistula also complicated pneumonectomy; division of the left recurrent laryngeal nerve in a further six probably contributed importantly to the severity of the pulmonary infection because of difficulty in clearing bronchial secretions. Death in convalescence after pneumonectomy was attributed to myocardial infarction in 22 patients. In 7 of these 22 patients there was a history of myocardial infarction—once in five and twice in two of them—in the 10 years which preceded pneumonectomy and in four others there was a history of angina of effort. In 19 other patients submitted to pneumonectomy who did not develop important post-operative complications, there was also a history of coronary thrombosis, in the preceding 10 years, and in 14 there was a history of angina. Of the 22 who died from myocardial infarction there occurred during operation in six an acute event associated with hypotension, believed at the time probably to represent myocardial infarction, confirmed within a few hours, electrocardiographically, as myocardial infarction, and terminating three to 10 days later in death. It has been the habit for many years in this Unit to make routinely before thoracotomy for any purpose in all patients over the age of 40 an electrocardiograph which serves as a basis for comparison with similar records made for whatever indication in convalescence, and this proved particularly useful in judging electrocardiographic change in those whose myocardial infarction developed during operation. Only three of the 22 patients who died from coronary thrombosis after pneumonectomy were younger than 50 years—the youngest was 41—and two of these three had had previous myocardial infarcts; the two oldest of the 22 were 70 and 71 years respectively. Pulmonary embolism accounted for death in 20 patients.

Death in five patients was related directly to surgical error; in one the pulmonary artery was divided with a ligature—an accident from which recovery was not made and subsequent to which it has been the habit always to control the pulmonary artery proximally with a clamp and, after division of the vessel, to secure the proximal cut end with a vascular stitch, a habit which has not been complicated in many hundreds of pneumonectomies, and one which has the additional advantage of allowing trainees to become accustomed to suturing large vessels; death in two patients occurred on the day of operation, in one because the ligature came off a pulmonary vein and in the other because the ligature came off the pulmonary artery; and death in two patients is recorded on the day of operation as the consequence of haemorrhage without the source of haemorrhage being specified.

Death in seven patients was the result of prolonged hypotension with a state of low cardiac output; management was with pressor agents, in some over many days; in three the cause of hypotension was not clear, at necropsy; in four there were suprarenal metastases.

Death in 14 patients had a vascular or cardiac cause—pulmonary venous thrombosis in one and pulmonary arterial thrombosis in another; a cerebrovascular accident in three; cor pulmonale in two; and congestive cardiac failure in seven.

One patient died from cerebral embolism at operation, the consequence of a tumour embolus dislodged into the left heart from a pulmonary vein occluded by tumour—an event surprisingly infrequent when the number of patients is considered in whom a nubbin of tumour is found to project into the left atrium. Three patients are recorded as having died from necrotising enteritis —a diagnosis made post-mortem but with reasoned and convincing ante-mortem clinical evidence—but nonetheless a diagnosis now rarely made, and one that seemed, for a period of a few years, to be made frequently.

Two patients died from contralateral spontaneous pneumothorax—a diagnosis difficult to make in a patient suddenly and acutely ill during convalescence from pneumonectomy, successfully made in two other patients who survived and in whom the pneumothorax was intubated, and its possibility an indication always to radiograph as a matter of urgency the chest of any patient inexplicably ill at any stage in convalescence from pneumonectomy.

Unsuspected hepatic metastases were found in 17 of 121 patients who died in convalescence after pneumonectomy. Suprarenal metastases were found in nine other patients—four of these have been mentioned above; small cerebral metastases were found in 11 patients—nine of these had hepatic or suprarenal metastases also. Glandular spread outwith the area cleared of glands at pneumonectomy was found in 42 patients who did not have other evidence of spread. Only 21 of 121 patients who died after pneumonectomy were found not to have evidence of tumour spread—necropsy could not be undertaken in 10 patients.

Of the 786 patients who survived pneumonectomy for bronchial carcinoma, 77 have died from causes not related to recurrence of tumour. Of the 77, 29 patients died either from coronary thrombosis or from acute coronary artery insufficiency complicating angina of effort. One of the 29 patients was a woman who did not smoke. At the time of pneumonectomy the youngest was 37, two were in the fifth decade, eight in the sixth, 12 in the seventh, and six in the eighth decade. There was a history of coronary thrombosis before pneumonectomy in five of the 29 patients in this group, and of these five three died less than six months after pneumonectomy, one two and one five years after pneumonectomy. Death from coronary artery disease in those submitted to pneumonectomy when they were in the eighth decade occurred in three in the second year after pneumonectomy, in two in the fourth year and in one in the eighth year after pneumonectomy. Atrial fibrillation complicated pneumonectomy in nine of this group of 29 patients. Of the whole group of 29 patients, five had died within a year of pneumonectomy, four more within two years, and a further nine survived less than five years; the remainder survived pneumonectomy by more than five years, three of them by more than 10 years. The resected tumour had been squamous in 22, in four of these with glandular metastases; undifferentiated in three; an adenocarcinoma in two; and mixed in two patients. In two patients who died from coronary artery insufficiency five and seven years, respectively, after pneumonectomy, the tumour had been in the left main bronchus and had extended to within 2 cm. of the main carina; in two further patients, both of whom died seven years after pneumonectomy, the left recurrent laryngeal nerve had been sacrificed in order to make more complete resection of mediastinal lymph glands shown histologically to be invaded by tumour.

Of the 77 patients who died from causes not related to tumour recurrence, 12, two of them women, died with cor pulmonale—two in the second year after pneumonectomy (a woman of 63 years, and a coal-miner of 58 years who did not smoke and who had, in addition, progressive massive fibrosis), and the remainder five to nine years after pneumonectomy. The tumour had been squamous in eight and undifferentiated in four; atrial fibrillation had developed in three during early convalescence; in one the tumour had been in the left main bronchus, and in one the left recurrent laryngeal nerve had been sacrificed.

Eleven men died, all of them four or more years after pneumonectomy, in congestive cardiac failure. The youngest was 46 years old at the time of operation, two were in the sixth decade, three in the seventh, and five in the eighth decade. Of those in the eighth decade at the time of pneumonectomy, two died four years later, one seven, one eight and one 12 years after pneumonectomy—in these bronchial carcinoma and pneumonectomy cannot reasonably be blamed for shortening life. Three of the 11 patients in this group developed atrial fibrillation early in convalescence; one had in addition to bronchial carcinoma, pulmonary tuberculosis; and in one an oesophageal leiomyoma was found incidentally at thoracotomy and was resected. The tumours in eight were squamous, in two adenocarcinomata and in one an undifferentiated carcinoma, called " oat-cell ".

Fifteen men died—eight within a year of pneumonectomy— from pulmonary infection, and in this group the fact of having been deprived of one lung almost certainly contributed importantly to death, but in none was there clinical evidence of metastases, and at necropsy in 12 evidence of tumour recurrence or metastases was not found. Three died in the second year after pneumonectomy, and the others four to nine years after operation. The youngest was 42 at the time of pulmonary resection, the oldest 72, and the others were in the sixth or seventh decade. One—who died four years after pneumonectomy, was one of the two patients who survived contralateral spontaneous pneumothorax after pneumonectomy. Another had been submitted to oesophago-gastrectomy for adenocarcinoma at the cardio-oesophageal junction two years before being subjected to pneumonectomy for squamous carcinoma—he died from aspiration pneumonia two years after pneumonectomy—a catastrophe almost certainly related to the fact that he had been deprived of the mechanism at the cardia which prevents reflux. Of those who died from pulmonary infection late after pneumonectomy, the tumour had been squamous in nine, undifferentiated in five and alveolar in one.

Of the remaining 10 patients who died from causes other than recurrence or metastases from bronchial carcinoma, five died from other tumours—all adenocarcinomata, one of the rectum, one of the colon, one at the pylorus, one in the stomach, and one at the oesophago-gastric junction—the pulmonary tumours in four having been squamous and in one undifferentiated. The second tumour was recognised three to nine years after pneumonectomy; in none was surgical management undertaken; all were over 55 years of age at the time of pneumonectomy and one was 70.

Five patients have yet to be accounted for from this group of 77; one died 10 years after pneumonectomy from a dissecting aortic aneurysm; one died four years after pneumonectomy from gastro-intestinal haemorrhage; one from miliary tuberculosis in the remaining lung a year after pneumonectomy; one from a cerebro-vascular accident four and a half years after pneumonectomy; and the last from peritonitis, the cause of which was never explained, nine months after pneumonectomy.

In this group of 77 patients there was evidence by necropsy of absence of tumour recurrence or metastases in 59; in the remainder—all of whom died more than three years after pneumonectomy—there was no clinical evidence of recurrence at the time of death, and on a chest radiograph, made in all within seven months of death, the appearances were normal after pneumonectomy.

In Chapter IV the results of pneumonectomy for bronchial carcinoma are discussed in relation to the histological type of the resected tumour. Of the 977 patients managed by pneumonectomy, 510 have died from metastases—107 within six months of operation, a further 141 within a year of resection, 119 more in the second year after resection, and the remainder three to 11 years after resection. All but two of the 35 patients with adenocarcinoma had died within five years of operation—whether or not glands were invaded at the time of pneumonectomy. The death rates, including operative mortality, for squamous and undifferentiated carcinoma, in the first three years after pneumonectomy are shown in Figure 3. At the end of three years—ignoring for the purpose of this calculation patients who had died from causes other than carcinoma after pneumonectomy—50 per cent of the total number of patients submitted to pneumonectomy for squamous carcinoma were alive, and 57 per cent of those who survived pneumonectomy for squamous carcinoma were alive; in comparison, only 31 per cent of the total number of patients submitted to pneumonectomy for undifferentiated carcinoma were alive, and 35 per cent of those who survived pneumonectomy for undifferentiated carcinoma were alive. In the fourth and subsequent years the death rate from metastases or recurrence after pneumonectomy for either squamous or undifferentiated carcinoma is very much less rapid, but deaths from metastases or recurrence occur even 12 years after pneumonectomy.

Of those 107 patients who died from metastases within six months of pneumonectomy, 44 died from cerebral metastases as the only clinical evidence of dissemination of tumour, and 15 other patients had cerebral metastases as well as other evidence of spread at the time of death. Osseous metastases, spinal in five, were clinically and radiographically obvious in 13 patients at the time of death; hepatic metastases in seven and pulmono-pulmonary metastases in five; lymphangitis carcinomatosa in two patients and clinically palpable suprarenal metastases in two others are recorded. In seven of the 107 patients in this group pneumonectomy had involved deliberate sacrifice of the left recurrent laryngeal nerve, and in two patients pneumonectomy had included resection of part of the chest wall. Unusual metastases included, in one patient who presented originally without symptoms and with an abnormal mass miniature chest radiograph, metastases in the lip, cheek, toes and skull, and in another patient a metastasis in the ischio-rectal fossa, which presented clinically as an ischio-rectal abscess.

Of the 141 patients who died six to 12 months after pneumonectomy, 38 died with cerebral metastases as the only clinical evidence of tumour dissemination, 14 with osseous metastases, including four with paraplegia, 13 with hepatic metastases, eight with pulmono-pulmonary metastases, five with mediastinal recurrence responsible for interruption of the left recurrent laryngeal nerve and external compression of the oesophagus, four with diffuse subcutaneous metastases and three with pleural metastases. In others, there were metastases in several sites including cervical lymph glands. In this group of patients the left recurrent nerve had been deliberately divided at pneumonectomy in six patients, three had never smoked, in three the resected lung contained active tuberculosis, and in four oesophageal displacement had been demonstrated at routine pre-operative investigation.

Of the 119 patients who died from metastases in the second year after pneumonectomy, 37 died with cerebral metastases as the only evidence of tumour spread—that is, within two years of pneumonectomy one in every three of 367 patients who died from metastases died with cerebral metastases as the only clinical evidence of tumour dissemination. It is only in the second year after pneumonectomy that obstruction of the superior vena cava was commonly recognised clinically—15 patients appeared with this as evidence of tumour recurrence; hepatic, pulmono-pulmonary and osseous metastases were common—equally distributed in 39 patients; in 14 patients mediastinal recurrence presented not only as obstruction of the superior vena cava but also as hoarseness of voice and dysphagia—separately or together; lymphangitis carcinomatosa, chest wall recurrence, scattered subcutaneous metastases in relation to the thoracotomy scar, and recurrence at the site of bronchial closure or in the trachea, and diffuse metastases are all recorded in this group. Amongst those who died from metastases in the second year after pneumonectomy were two of the youngest patients—a woman of 25 years submitted to pneumonectomy for an undifferentiated carcinoma, who was delivered of a normal child 10 months later and died 14 months after pneumonectomy; and a woman of 22 years, also with an undifferentiated carcinoma, who died 18 months after pneumonectomy. Three of the patients who died in the second year after pneumonectomy had been shown to have active tuberculosis in the resected lung, and one had progressive massive fibrosis; the left recurrent laryngeal nerve had been divided deliberately in three patients in this group.

Among those who died of metastases later than two years after pneumonectomy, there were fewer with cerebral metastases, but this, as a cause of death, is recorded as late as five years after pneumonectomy without other evidence of tumour from which cerebral dissemination could have occurred. Pulmono-pulmonary metastases and lymphangitis carcinomatosa were recognised nine to 12 years after pneumonectomy; obstruction of the superior vena cava was commonplace three to eight years after pneumonectomy; malignant pericarditis as the cause of death was recorded eighteen times two to eight years after pneumonectomy. An isolated renal metastasis which presented with haematuria and was recognised as a metastasis only after nephrectomy was managed in this way in five patients. None survived nephrectomy by more than three years, and other evidence of metastasis was apparent clinically in all for at least eight months before death.

At the time when this survey was completed, 31 patients were alive after pneumonectomy, but had clinical or radiological evidence of metastasis. Of these 31 patients 25 were alive two to four years after pneumonectomy. The evidence of metastasis or recurrence was obstruction of the superior vena cava (four patients); left recurrent laryngeal nerve palsy (three patients); others were recognised as having cervical lymph-glandular metastases (six patients), recurrence at the site of bronchial closure (two patients), recurrence of tumour in the wound, in the form of multiple subcutaneous tumours but not in the thoracotomy scar (two patients), pulmono-pulmonary metastases (five patients), and cerebral metastases (three patients). Those in this group of 25 with symptoms possibly remediable by irradiation had been or were being irradiated. There were six patients alive nine to 12 years after pneumonectomy in whom tumour had recurred—in four at the bronchial stump eight to 11 years after pneumonectomy, and all were well nine to 12 years after pneumonectomy, the recurrence having been irradiated; and in two with an unusual history. One patient was alive, well and working normally 11 years after pneumonectomy and 10 years after a metastasis had been resected from the omentum; he presented a year after pneumonectomy with abdominal pain and a mass in the left hypochondrium; the mass was resected and was shown to be a metastasis the size of a tennis ball, wrapped in omentum, and not attached to any other structure. The last patient alive with known recurrence of tumour was well 10 years after pneumonectomy and five years after resection of an apparently isolated cerebellar metastasis.

In Chapter IV the histology of the resected tumour is related to survival time in the 238 patients known to be alive and well and without clinically or radiographically recognised metastasis at the time of completing this survey. The six who survived longest were submitted to pneumonectomy more than 16 years ago—two for adenocarcinoma (these are the only two patients alive after pneumonectomy for adenocarcinoma, and both would now have been managed by lobectomy); and four for undifferentiated carcinoma. Of those alive, 25 per cent had glandular metastases at the time of pneumonectomy.

The outcome of surgical management by pneumonectomy of 35 patients with adenocarcinoma, and a further eight patients with mixed tumour which included adenocarcinoma, can be summarised: seven died as a direct consequence of operation; five died one to eight years after operation, from causes other than recurrence of tumour: 15 died of cerebral metastases, 13 of them within a year of operation; 13 died from tumour recurrence or metastases other than cerebral, most more than a year after operation; and three are alive, two 16 years after pneumonectomy and one in whom the histological appearances of the bronchoscopic biopsy were those of undifferentiated carcinoma and of the operative specimen those of adenocarcinoma, 14 years after pneumonectomy.

Some of those at present alive more than two but less than five years after pneumonectomy will almost certainly die from metastases, as will some of those alive more than five years after pneumonectomy and apparently entirely well at the present time. But of 977 patients submitted to pneumonectomy for carcinoma, 238 (24 per cent) are alive at the present time without clinical or radiographic evidence of metastases, and all of them more than two years after pneumonectomy. Of 786 patients submitted to pneumonectomy more than five years ago 157 (20 per cent) are alive and well, without evidence of metastases. Cognisance is not taken here of patients who died more than five years after pneumonectomy but not from the consequence of metastases or tumour recurrence. Similar results are recorded by others.[1, 2, 3]

[1] Ogilvie C., Harris, L. H., Meecham, J. & Ryder, G. (1963). Ten years after pneumonectomy for carcinoma. *Br. med. J.,* **1,** 1111.
[2] Belcher, J. R. & Anderson, R. (1965). Surgical treatment of carcinoma of the bronchus. *Br. med. J.* **1,** 948.
[3] Bignall, J. R., Martin, M. & Smithers, D. W. (1967). Survival in 6,086 cases of bronchial carcinoma. *Lancet,* **1,** 1067.

III. MANAGEMENT BY LOBECTOMY

Bronchial carcinoma in 470 patients (12 per cent) was managed by lobectomy—by the resection of a single lobe in 318 patients; by the resection of two lobes in 91 patients; and by resection of a lobe, or two lobes, with part of the stem bronchus (" sleeve " resection[1]) in 61 patients. The anatomical distribution of resected lobes is shown in Tables XXI and XXII. The commonest

TABLE XXI

Lobectomy (470)

	Right	Left	Total	Male	Female
One lobe	128	190	318	289	29
Two lobes	91		91	84	7
Sleeve re-section	57 (2 lobes in 5)	4	61	58	3
Total	276	194	470	431	39

TABLE XXII

Lobectomy (470)

Right		Left			
		Deaths			Deaths
Upper lobe	75	8	Upper lobe	118	6
Upper lobe with sleeve	52	—	Upper lobe with sleeve	4	—
Middle lobe	11	1			
Lower lobe	42	4	Lower lobe	72	7
Middle & upper	23	2			
Middle & upper with sleeve	5	—			
Middle & lower	68	7			
Total	276	22	Total	194	13

resection was left upper lobectomy—in 118 patients. Right-sided resections (276) were more numerous than left-sided resections (194) because of the possibility on the right of resecting pairs of lobes—middle lobectomy alone contributed negligibly to the total.

The distribution of tumours—whether peripheral or central—is shown in Table XXIII. Where a single lobe was resected, the tumour was peripheral in five of every six resections undertaken. Where two lobes were resected or a " sleeve " resection was undertaken, the tumours were more commonly central than peripheral. The commonest indication for double lobectomy was a tumour

[1] Price-Thomas, Sir Clement (1956). Conservative resection of the bronchial tree. *Jl R. Coll. Surg. Edinb.*, **1**, 169.

TABLE XXIII

Lobectomy

	Peripheral	*Central*	*Total*
One lobe	265	53	318
Two lobes	33	58	91
Sleeve resection	4	57	61
Total	302 (25 deaths)	168 (10 deaths)	470 (35 deaths)

visible in the right stem bronchus, usually distal to the origin of the middle bronchus—in these circumstances the middle lobe was resected with the lower lobe in order that the length of stem bronchus called alternatively " lower part of right main " or " intermediate " could be included in the resection to clear more widely the tumour, with stem bronchus closure at the lower lip of the right upper bronchus. Middle and upper lobectomy together were undertaken when the tumour—usually of peripheral type—transgressed the transverse fissure or grew in anatomical circumstances which made middle and upper lobes for practical purposes one, with absence of the transverse fissure. " Sleeve " resection was most often undertaken for a tumour which was bronchoscopically visible in the right upper bronchus, and only four " sleeve " resections of a total of 61 were undertaken for a peripheral type of tumour.

The histological range in this group of 470 lobectomies has been outlined in Chapter IV. Squamous tumours were the most common (65 per cent); undifferentiated tumours (18 per cent) and adenocarcinomata (15 per cent) were of nearly equal frequency, and the number of undifferentiated tumours managed by lobectomy is very much smaller than the number found irresectable and the number managed by pneumonectomy: 66 per cent of undifferentiated tumours were unsuitable for any form of surgical management. Where the cell type found at bronchoscopic biopsy differed from that of the operative specimen or mediastinal glands, one of the cell types was, in all the 15 instances, of squamous carcinoma.

Age at the time of lobectomy is shown in Figure 10. Of the 470 patients managed in this way, 39 (8 per cent) were women. The graphic pattern of age as shown in Figure 10 is not significantly different from that which shows the age distribution in the series as a whole (Figs. 4-7), but in comparison with Figure 9, which illustrates the age distribution of patients managed by pneumonectomy, more patients over the age of 70 are suitable for management of bronchial carcinoma by lobectomy than pneumonectomy. Two women and 33 men died as a direct consequence of operation—an operative mortality of 7 per cent. Operative mortality in relation to age is shown in Table XIX, and it is clear that the operative mortality increases with age. The operative mortality in those younger than 65 is 4·5 per cent and in those 65 years or older is 14 per cent, while in those 70 years or older the operative mortality is 22 per cent.

71

Although left upper lobectomy was the operation most commonly under-taken, right upper lobectomy was the operation with the highest individual operative death rate—eight of 75 patients submitted to right upper lobectomy died, and six of 118 submitted to left upper lobectomy. None of the patients submitted to " sleeve " resection died. Of the 35 who died after operation, 14 died from pulmonary embolism, and 15 from pulmonary infection and pulmonary insufficiency. Death from pulmonary insufficiency after pulmonary resection seems to occur only when superadded pulmonary infection becomes uncontrolled. Of the remaining six patients who died after lobectomy, one died in congestive cardiac failure and one from supra-renal apoplexy, two died from coronary thrombosis, one from necrotising enteritis, and one from massive gastro-intestinal haemorrhage a week after a perforated duodenal ulcer had been closed at laparotomy—laparotomy having been undertaken a fortnight after lobectomy.

Of those who survived operation, 37 patients have died from causes not related to tumour recurrence—two of these 37 were women, and three of these patients had never smoked. Eight patients all of whom were older than 60 years died in the first 12 months after discharge from hospital—three from coronary artery disease, two from pulmonary infection and cardiac failure together, one from nephritis, one from cerebral thrombosis and one from gastro-intestinal haemorrhage. Two patients died in the second year after lobectomy—both from coronary thrombosis—and four in the fourth year after lobectomy—two from pulmonary infection, and two in congestive cardiac failure; one of these last-mentioned was aged 75 at the time of death. Twenty-three patients have died five to 12 years after lobectomy from causes clearly established on clinical grounds and in 13 substantiated by necropsy evidence as unrelated to tumour recurrence. The oldest of these was 84 at the time of death, and two were 79. One of these last-mentioned two died five years after lobectomy and the other 11 years after lobectomy and nine years after resection of a gastric carcinoma of histological type different from that of the resected pulmonary tumour.

In Chapter IV the results of resection are assessed in relation to the histological type of the resected tumour. Of the 470 patients in whom bronchial carcinoma was managed by lobectomy, 171 have died from metastases—14 within six months of resection, a further 43 within a year of resection, 55 more in the second year after resection, and the remainder three to nine years after resection. The mortality from metastases from adenocarcinoma seems dispro-portionately high in the second year after resection.

Seven patients are alive with metastases, all more than four years after resection. Two have slowly growing pulmonary shadows presumed to be pulmono-pulmonary metastases, recognised three and four years after resection, respectively. In both the metastases grow little each year and the patients remain symptomless, one two and one three years after first recognition of the multiple pulmonary shadows. Two patients have peripheral cavitated shadows and have been shown to have tumour cells in the sputum. It is presumed that these cavitated isolated shadows are caused by pulmono-pulmonary metastases, but since they are single shadows, they may represent new primary tumours. Both these patients had squamous tumours, are declining slowly, and are unsuitable on the grounds of dyspnoea for any further operation and for radiotherapy. They have survived their original resection by seven and fifteen years respectively. One patient has osseous metastases five years after lobectomy and has been irradiated with relief of pain; his survival is unlikely to be prolonged. Three patients have presented seven to 10 years after lobectomy with a pulmonary tumour, visible at bronchoscopy, in a bronchus on the side opposite to that on which lobectomy was undertaken; in each instance the histological features of the new tumour are similar to those of the original—all are squamous. If these patients had not had a previous lobectomy, the radiographic and bronchoscopic appearances related to the contralateral tumour now present would be accepted as those of primary bronchial carcinoma rather than carcinoma which has presented in a bronchus the consequence of bronchial erosion from mediastinal glands. These three tumours may therefore represent new primary tumours rather than metastases. All have been irradiated; one patient is alive three years after irradiation and 11 years after lobectomy.

In Chapter IV the histology of the resected tumour is related to survival time in the 220 patients known to be alive and well and without clinical or radiographically recognisable metastases at the present time. The longest to survive was submitted to lobectomy for adenocarcinoma 15 years ago, at a time when lobectomy was rarely undertaken for bronchial carcinoma or for a peripheral pulmonary lesion without pre-operative histological confirmation of the diagnosis of carcinoma but which could reasonably only be called a carcinoma. Survival for five or 10 years after lobectomy for a squamous or undifferentiated tumour with glandular metastases is not uncommon. Of those who have survived lobectomy by more than six years, 15 are over 70 years of age at the present time, and a further five are over 80 years; lobectomy in these patients appears to have had little detrimental effect on longevity.

Some of those at present alive more than two but less than five years after lobectomy will almost certainly die from metastases, as will some of those alive more than five years after lobectomy and apparently entirely well at the present time. Of 470 patients submitted to lobectomy for carcinoma 220 (47 per cent) are alive at the present time, without clinical or radiographic evidence of metastases, and all of them are alive more than two years after lobectomy. Of 351 patients submitted to lobectomy more than five years ago 134 (38 per cent) are alive and well, without evidence of metastases. Cognisance is not taken, here, of patients who died more than five years after operation, but not from the consequence of metastases or recurrence of tumour.

IV. MANAGEMENT BY SEGMENTAL RESECTION

Segmental resection was undertaken in 17 patients. At no time in the period under discussion was segmental resection regarded as an acceptable alternative to, say, lobectomy in the management of established bronchial carcinoma, and the circumstances in which segmental resection was undertaken in these 17 patients were unusual.

Of the 17 patients eight were older than 65 years—four of these older than 70. The youngest patient was 39 years. All but one were men. In all, the tumour was peripheral in type and the appearances at bronchoscopy were normal. The tumours were on the right in eight and on the left in nine patients. In seven patients the segment resected was an apical segment of an upper lobe and in another seven an apical segment of a lower lobe; in two the lingular segment was resected and in one a segment of the middle lobe. Presentation in five symptomless patients was with an abnormal chest radiograph made for routine purposes and in one patient presentation was with the symptoms of hypertrophic pulmonary osteoarthropathy. The peripheral spherical pulmonary shadow in three patients measured 1 cm. in transverse diameter; in seven other patients the peripheral pulmonary shadow measured less than 1·5 cm. and in five other patients less than 2 cm. in transverse diameter; in only two patients was the pulmonary opacity greater than 2 cm. in diameter. In 12 patients the tumour was squamous in type, in one undifferentiated, and in four patients the tumour was an adenocarcinoma. In three patients the resected segment included a healed tuberculous lesion in very close proximity to the tumour; in two patients there were two separate tumours in the same segment, one smaller than the other, and not separately recognised tomographically, and interpreted as a tuberculous focus with a satellite lesion in close proximity at operation: in two patients the tumour was of calcific hardness.

The reasons for management of bronchial carcinoma by segmental resection in these 17 patients were: (a) interpretation by palpation of the lesion in seven patients as tuberculous—on the grounds of hardness, related scarring or multiplicity of nodules; (b) separation of the resected segment from neighbouring segments by an anatomically complete fissure in five patients, in four of whom the apical segment of a lower lobe and in one of whom the lingular segment were resected; in these the lesion was recognised as most probably a carcinoma, but it was judged as effective to manage the tumour by segmental resection as by lobectomy; (c) severe limitation of respiratory reserve in five patients, in whom thoracotomy was undertaken with a view to doing the most limited resection possible to establish the diagnosis of carcinoma, and in whom it had been decided before operation that a resection greater than lobectomy would not be undertaken.

Of the 17 patients in whom bronchial carcinoma was managed by segmental resection, one died from respiratory failure as a direct result of operation—one of the five in whom respiratory function was severely limited. Five patients are alive—two of these five years after segmental resection, one six years and two eight years after operation—and in three of these five segmental resection was undertaken because of completeness of anatomical separation of the resected segment from adjacent lung. Of the five long survivors the tumour in two was an adenocarcinoma and in three a squamous carcinoma. Two still work as miners at the coal face. Eleven patients have died, eight of these from metastases and three from causes apparently unrelated to bronchial carcinoma. Two patients died from metastases within a year of operation, four in the third post-operative year, one in the fifth and one in the seventh. Two patients died from coronary artery disease two years after operation and one died 18 months after operation in the following circumstances: left apical segmental resection had been undertaken in the belief that the lesion was tuberculous and when the histological report of carcinoma was received further treatment was by radiotherapy to the area from which the segment had been removed; nine months later he was ill with severe pulmonary infection and either an abscess in the left upper lobe or a localised left upper empyema; he failed to improve on conservative management and the loculus of pus was drained anteriorly by rib resection; a large pulmonary slough was removed at this operation, and subsequent bronchography demonstrated communication between the left upper bronchus and the large, static left upper pleural space with its anterior parietal drain; radiotherapy was judged responsible for sphacelation of most of what remained of the left upper lobe after apical segmental resection; continued deterioration in health and recurrent contralateral aspiration pneumonia prompted injudicious closure of the left upper space by thoracoplasty, in convalescence from which he died; metastases were not found at necropsy. Radiotherapy was not used in other patients in this group of 17 until there was evidence of recurrence of tumour.

From the small number of segmental resections undertaken it can only be said that this operation undertaken in the management of bronchial carcinoma is followed by long survival in a proportion of patients not noticeably different from that which follows resection of greater extent for tumours of the same relatively small size. Since in none of the patients managed by segmental resection were hilar glands resected for histological examination, and since none of the operative notes contain specific comment on the presence or absence of such glands, it is not possible to relate survival to the absence of hilar glandular invasion, although this remains a reasonable assumption. In three patients who died with metastases there was radiographic evidence before death and histological evidence after necropsy of local recurrence of tumour. In one of these patients local recurrence became radiographically evident in the fourth year after segmental resection for squamous carcinoma, and death was delayed a further three years by irradiation. Death was related to distant metastases or mediastinal growth of tumour in the remainder who died with metastases—hepatic metastases without local recurrence in two, obstruction of the superior vena cava in two, and interruption of the left recurrent laryngeal nerve in one. Survival time, and the pattern of emergence of metastatic tumour or recurrence of tumour at the site of resection or in the mediastinum are therefore also not noticeably different in those managed by segmental resection from those which follow resection of greater extent.

VII

The Influence of Presentation Without Symptoms and With an Abnormal Chest Radiograph, on Results of Management

SUMMARY

Of 4,000 patients with bronchial carcinoma, 192 (4·8 per cent) presented without symptoms and with an abnormal chest radiograph made for an unrelated purpose. Patients in this group were more often suitable for surgical management of bronchial carcinoma than were those who presented because of symptoms, but not all were suitable, and in some there was clinical evidence of tumour dissemination.

The number of patients with peripheral tumours was substantially higher and the number of patients with undifferentiated tumours substantially lower than the series as a whole. Only a third had central tumours. The resection undertaken was a lobectomy in 70, pneumonectomy in 55, and in five, segmental resection. Operative mortality and the rate of irresectability at exploratory thoracotomy (both 5 per cent) were lower and the long survival rate (40 per cent) for all resections was higher than in the rest of the series.

O F 4,000 patients with bronchial carcinoma 192 were investigated because they were found at mass radiography—made for an unrelated routine purpose—to have an abnormal chest radiograph. Facts which relate to some of these patients have been presented elsewhere.[1] A further large number of patients came for investigation with an abnormal film from a mass radiography unit, but these patients had been referred for radiography, usually by a general practitioner, because of respiratory or other symptoms and are not included in the figure of 192. Of the 192, 17 were women, of whom the youngest was 35, three were in the fifth decade, five in the sixth, six in the seventh and the two oldest were 72 and 79 years respectively. The youngest of the 175 men were 32 and 33 years respectively; 29 men (16·5 per cent) were younger than 50 and 25 (15 per cent) were older than 69, the oldest being 80 years; 120 men were in the sixth or seventh decade, and all but 15 of these were older than 55 years.

The pulmonary tumour in these 192 patients was associated with an abnormality at bronchoscopy in only a third, while in two-thirds (128 patients)

---

[1] Seiler, H. E., Welstead, A. G. & Williamson, J. (1958). Report on Edinburgh X-ray campaign, 1958. *Tubercle*, **39**, 339.

the tumours were peripheral in type; in these patients the bronchoscopic appearances were normal. The histological features were those of squamous carcinoma in 107, of which 67 were peripheral tumours; in 45 the tumour was called undifferentiated (" oat cell " in three of these) and 22 of these were peripheral; in 15 the tumour was an adenocarcinoma, peripheral in all but one; in four the tumour was an alveolar-cell carcinoma, peripheral and an isolated, well-defined opacity in all; in 21 patients, all with peripheral shadows, a histological diganosis was not achieved, but collateral evidence made the diagnosis of carcinoma the only tenable one.

Of the 192 patients 151 smoked cigarettes and seven were pipe smokers; four used to smoke cigarettes but had not smoked for 16, 15, 11 and five years respectively; the smoking habits of 19 patients are not recorded, and 11 did not smoke. Of the eleven who did not smoke, nine were women, in three of whom the tumour was an adenocarcinoma, in three others of whom the tumour was an undifferentiated carcinoma, and in the last three the diagnosis of squamous carcinoma, " oat cell " carcinoma and alveolar-cell carcinoma was made, respectively. The two non-smoking men had squamous tumours.

Of the 15 patients with an adenocarcinoma one, in whom a cervical gland contained tumour, was not treated surgically; he died six months after irradiation. The others were managed surgically, 12 by lobectomy, one by pneumonectomy and one by segmental resection. Pneumonectomy was required in the only patient with a central adenocarcinoma, and he died with cerebral metastases just short of three years after pneumonectomy. The patient submitted to segmental resection died two years after operation with hepatic metastases and without residual tumour in the chest. Of those submitted to lobectomy four are alive—nine, seven, four and two years after resection respectively; one, a woman, who did not smoke, returned seven years after lobectomy with a new ipsilateral shadow, management of which was by completion of pneumonectomy, and the tumour was now called an alveolar-cell carcinoma, differing widely in histological appearance from the original lesion—she remains well; and seven have died, all from metastases, two four years, one three years, and the others 12-20 months after operation. Of the two other non-smokers, one is alive two years after lobectomy and one died three years after lobectomy with cerebral metastases.

Omitting the patient mentioned above whose second tumour was an alveolar-cell carcinoma, there were four patients with alveolar-cell tumours, of whom one, a non-smoking woman, is alive seven years after lobectomy, the second is alive seven years after pneumonectomy (in his case mediastinal glands were invaded), and two were alive five and three years, respectively, after lobectomy.

The tumour in 45 patients was an undifferentiated carcinoma. In ten of these management was other than surgical, in two because of a limited respiratory reserve, in one because of associated myocardial disease, and in seven because of evidence of tumour dissemination—cervical lymph-glandular metastases in four, nodular hepatomegaly in one, and displacement of the barium filled oesophagus and phrenic paresis in two. All had died within a year of investigation.

One patient with an undifferentiated tumour was submitted to thoracotomy and the tumour was shown widely to invade the mediastinum; resection was not undertaken and he died seven months later. In the remaining 34 a resection was undertaken—lobectomy in 16, in three of these with part of the stem bronchus, and pneumonectomy in 18. Of those submitted only to lobectomy, one died 12 years after operation from coronary insufficiency and without necropsy evidence of residual tumour, and five were alive, two seven years after operation, one five years and two three years after operation. Both those alive seven years after resection had mediastinal glandular metastases, and in one of these who did not smoke the tumour was called " oat-cell ". There were two operative deaths after lobectomy, one from necrotising enteritis, and one from suprarenal apoplexy; and five patients have died from metastases, all within two years of operation—two of those who died from metastases had mediastinal glandular metastases and three did not.

Only three of the 18 patients submitted to pneumonectomy for an undifferentiated carcinoma are alive—two eight years after operation, and in one of these the phrenic nerve was deliberately sacrificed at thoracotomy to allow of a wider resection of an area of invaded pericardium, and one two years after operation; neither had mediastinal glandular invasion. There were two operative deaths after pneumonectomy, both from a combination of respiratory infection and lack of respiratory reserve. Thirteen patients have died from metastases after pneumonectomy in this group, seven within a year of operation, four others in the second year after operation, and two four years after operation. Nine of the 13 had mediastinal glandular metastases, including the two longest survivors who died with metastases. One who died in the second year did not smoke, and another was submitted to resection in the knowledge that there was fluoroscopic evidence of slight displacement of the barium filled oesophagus—displacement confirmed at thoracotomy to be by glands invaded by tumour.

The tumour in 107 patients, who presented with an abnormal mass miniature or other routine radiograph, was squamous in type. Of the 107 patients, five declined treatment, and all had died within 18 months of investigation, four within eight months. Poor respiratory reserve in one patient precluded surgical management, and he is alive five years after irradiation, having survived a spontaneous pneumothorax on the side opposite to that irradiated three years ago. In three patients displacement of the barium filled oesophagus was accepted as a contra-indication to surgical management; the tumour was irradiated and all died within six months. In four patients the tumour encroached on the main carina or the trachea; the tumour was irradiated and three died within six months; the fourth is alive seven years after irradiation. Three patients had other evidence of tumour dissemination—an invaded cervical gland in one, nodular hepatomegaly in another, and pleural invasion proved by biopsy at thoracoscopy in the third—and all died within six months. Two patients died from coronary artery disease during investigation.

Of the 107 patients with squamous tumours 89 were managed surgically— 42 by lobectomy, three of these with " sleeve " resection, 36 by pneumonectomy, four by segmental resection and in seven the tumour was irresectable. Of those managed only by lobectomy, 19 are alive and well—three five years after operation, three seven years, four eight years, three nine years, one 11 years and one 14 years after operation, and four less than five years but more than two years after operation. Five of the primary tumours in these 19 patients were less than 4 cm. in diameter and the smallest was 1 cm. in diameter. In three, including two who are now long survivors, mediastinal glands were invaded, and one, now alive for nine years, developed pulmonary tuberculosis, of which he has been cured by chemotherapy, three years after lobectomy for carcinoma. Three other patients who are alive after lobectomy have evidence of tumour recurrence—one five years after operation, with osseous metastases; one seven years after operation with a squamous tumour in the opposite main bronchus, now irradiated, and this may have been a second primary tumour; and the third with tumour cells in the sputum and a peripheral cavitated pulmonary opacity seven years after lobectomy, in whom management has been neither by resection nor by irradiation because of dyspnoea, and he is alive nearly eight years after lobectomy. Twelve patients have died from metastases following lobectomy for squamous carcinoma, three within a year of operation, five within two years of operation, and four in the fourth year after resection. Only one of these 12 patients was shown to have mediastinal glandular metastases at operation. Of the 39 patients with squamous tumours managed only by lobectomy, five remain for discussion. Of these, one died on the first post-operative day from respiratory insufficiency, one died eight weeks after operation from massive gastro-intestinal haemorrhage, the third died six months after operation from pulmonary infection and at necropsy had one small hepatic metastasis, and the last two died four and five years after operation, respectively, one in congestive cardiac failure and the other from a cerebral vascular accident, neither with evidence of metastasis at necropsy.

Of the three patients submitted to lobectomy and resection of part of the stem bronchus, two are alive seven and eight years after resection, respectively, and the third died 20 months after resection, having been irradiated, a year after resection, for superior vena caval obstruction.

Segmental resection in four patients has been followed by survival for eight years in two, in one of whom the limited resection was undertaken because of a poor respiratory reserve, and in the other because the tumour lay in the lingular segment which was separated from the rest of the left upper lobe by an almost complete fissure, and a more extensive resection seemed pointless. The other two have died, one five years after segmental resection and three years after irradiation for local recurrence, and the second 26 months after resection from hepatic metastases without local recurrence.

Of 36 patients submitted to pneumonectomy for squamous carcinoma found at mass radiography, seven are alive and well, one three years after operation, two six years, and one each at 7, 8, 10, and 11 years after operation—one, the eight-year survivor, having had mediastinal glandular metastases. Four other patients are alive with metastases—one with paralysis of the left recurrent laryngeal nerve, and one with an invaded neck gland, in both evidence of spread having developed a year after operation, and both alive after irradiation two years after operation; one with obstruction of the superior vena cava, relieved by irradiation, three years after operation, and the last with recurrence in the scar 16 months after operation.

Of 36 patients submitted to pneumonectomy 18 have died from metastases, four within a year of operation, seven in the second post-operative year, and all within three years of operation. In eight of these patients mediastinal glands were invaded. Five patients have died from causes other than metastases—four from coronary thrombosis two, three, six and 11 years after pneumonectomy, respectively, and the fifth from a cerebro-vascular accident four and a half years after pneumonectomy. The patient who died from coronary thrombosis 11 years after pneumonectomy had been found to have a peripheral pulmonary shadow when his chest was radiographed during convalescence from gastrectomy for ulcer, but he declined further investigation. He returned for advice when, 18 months later, he developed pain, and the pulmonary shadow had increased considerably in size and was associated with erosion laterally of the second to fourth ribs. Pneumonectomy and resection of part of the chest wall were undertaken. In this patient, therefore, the tumour was known to be present for 18 months before it was resected, and yet survival was prolonged and death was from a cause other than metastases.

There were two operative deaths after pneumonectomy, both from pulmonary insufficiency aggravated by post-operative pulmonary infection.

Seven patients with squamous carcinoma were submitted to thoracotomy and found to have tumours the extent of which either precluded resection or made this pointless. One died on the ninth post-operative day—in him cardiac invasion precluded resection; the others died 8-19 months after exploration, which in all was followed by irradiation.

Of the three patients with squamous tumours who did not smoke, two are alive, seven and nine years after lobectomy, respectively, and both had mediastinal glandular metastases at operation; one also had active pulmonary tuberculosis at the time of lobectomy.

Of 192 patients who presented without new respiratory symptoms and because of an abnormal mass miniature radiograph, a histological diagnosis was not achieved in 21, in whom management was other than by thoracotomy. Of the 21 patients, 10 declined treatment; all were over 60 years and the oldest was 80. In seven of the 10 a peripheral shadow was observed to grow from the time of first observation to death, 10 to 27 months later, and death in three of the seven patients was with cerebral metastases. Contact with the other three was lost. The most rapid growth of the shadow was from 2 to 11 cm. in diameter in eight months, and the slowest growth was from 3 to 5 cm. in 19 months.

Of the 21 managed other than surgically, respiratory function in seven was so poor that exploratory thoracotomy was precluded as a form of management, and only three of the seven were acceptable to the radiotherapists for treatment, so limited was their reserve. All died within a year; four of the seven were miners submitted to routine yearly chest radiography; all were over 65; in only one was death clearly from tumour, while in the others, from available information, pulmonary infection and coronary insufficiency appear to have been the terminal episodes. The four who remain from this group of 21 all had evidence of mediastinal invasion—displacement at fluoroscopy of the barium filled oesophagus and/or phrenic paresis. In all the tumour was irradiated and all died at home within six months of investigation and without necropsy.

From this analysis of 192 patients referred because of an abnormal mass miniature or other routine chest radiograph some facts emerge. There is no significant difference in the age distribution of this group of patients from that of the series as a whole. The number of peripheral tumours is significantly higher and the number of undifferentiated tumours significantly lower than in the series as a whole; peripheral squamous tumours, often of small size, and adenocarcinomata were relatively common. The number of patients submitted to thoracotomy was also significantly higher—only 50 (26 per cent), of whom 10 declined thoracotomy, were not managed surgically. Resection was frustrated in eight patients and completed in 134, of whom seven died as the direct consequence of thoracotomy —an operative mortality and a rate of irresectability each of about 5 per cent— figures significantly lower than in the series as a whole. Long survival, amongst those who withstood resection, was 40 per cent—again higher than in the series as a whole. And apart from these statistical facts, some general facts relevant to the use of mass miniature and other routine films can be stated.

Because so many of the symptomless patients who present with an abnormal mass miniature radiograph have a pulmonary tumour which is peripheral, small, slow-growing and squamous, longer average survival in this group is to be expected, even if there is delay in their referral for a surgical opinion—and this there often was when tuberculosis was still a common disease. But it is totally unjustifiable to condone delay in referral for a surgical opinion on the ground that little material difference in ultimate result can be demonstrated. The resection of a tuberculoma or other lesion not certainly best treated surgically is infinitely preferable to delay in the surgical management of a pulmonary carcinoma.

The circumstances of mass and routine chest radiography are varied. In this series, some two-fifths of the patients who presented with an abnormal chest radiograph, and without new respiratory symptoms, were submitted to radiography during one of a series of mass radiography campaigns in the South-East Region of Scotland, most of them during 1957 and 1958. Routine

6

surveys of office and factory staff, of miners by the National Coal Board, and routine films of patients previously treated for tuberculosis, or of patients about to be subjected to elective surgery other than thoracic, constituted the commonest sources of abnormal films. Prospective emigrants and symptomless persons seeking to insure themselves presented occasionally with abnormal routine films.

Those patients who declined treatment offered an opportunity, not justifiable in any other circumstances, of observing radiographically the varied rate of growth of pulmonary carcinoma, and the time interval between the recognition of a peripheral shadow and the development of metastases and symptoms. Survival time from operation in a small group of patients who declined the advice offered when first they presented with an abnormal routine film but who accepted surgical management when they developed symptoms could be compared with survival time in those without symptoms who accepted surgical management, and in those who presented for the first time with symptoms. The number of patients in the first group is too small, however, to permit any statement other than that survival time varied over the entire range from long survival with ultimate death without metastases to inoperability with rapid decline from metastases despite irradiation.

Some hazards are associated with routine radiography for whatever purpose. Observer error in the interpretation of routine miniature films has been accurately assessed, and the incidence of error is not high. Notwithstanding when a patient previously radiographed for routine purposes presents with respiratory symptoms or with a second film made for similar routine purposes, and the original film, passed as normal, is scrutinised with the knowledge gained from recognition of an abnormality in the later film, a similar abnormality in the earlier film is often recognised. This can be of the utmost value in reaching a decision on management, in making more likely the diagnosis of a chronic inflammatory lesion such as tuberculosis, in assessing the rate of natural growth and, thereby, the prognosis of malignant tumours, and in establishing the fact of growth of other lesions such as chondro-adenomata. Furthermore, a patient routinely radiographed at arbitrary intervals—say yearly—who develops respiratory symptoms such as haemoptysis in the interval between radiographs is inclined to ignore these symptoms in the knowledge that a recent film has been passed as normal and another film will be made in the not too distant future. Thus, a miner became hoarse two months after a routine film had been made—an abnormal hilar shadow was, in retrospect, present in this film—was reassured by his general practitioner on the ground of a normal radiographic report, and did not seek advice again until eight months later when he developed obstruction of the superior vena cava. Five patients are known to have tolerated haemoptysis for 7-11 months because this symptom developed in the interval between routine films. But these are unusual examples of possible hazards of routine radiography, the overall advantages of which have been clearly shown.

Many patients are found by chest radiography for a pulmonary complication after an elective surgical procedure other than thoracic, to have a pulmonary lesion other than the acute post-operative one and possibly related to its development. There can never be any justification for failing to make a chest radiograph before any elective surgical procedure in an adult. Where a thoracic surgical unit exists in close relation to general surgical charges and the opportunity for education is taken, 15-20 patients will be found in any one year in general surgical wards to have surgical pulmonary lesions—a strong argument in favour of close collaboration between the branches of surgery and against the isolation of special units in peripheral hospitals.

In the group of 192 patients who were found to have bronchial carcinoma on routine radiography are not included 59 patients who presented for mass radiography because of symptoms other than respiratory. These symptoms include sudden difficulty experienced in the control of previously well-managed diabetes, loss of weight, dyspepsia, angina pectoris, and so on.

VIII

The Incidence of Pulmonary Resection Undertaken with a Provisional and Later Unsubstantiated Diagnosis of Bronchial Carcinoma

SUMMARY

Over a 15-year period, when frozen section examination was not regularly available, 918 patients with peripheral pulmonary lesions, the routine preliminary investigation of which did not provide a diagnosis, were managed aggressively—by a diagnostic pulmonary resection which, before 1954, was, in some patients, of the magnitude of pneumonectomy, but after that date, was never more extensive than lobectomy and often no more than segmental resection. In 756 patients (82 per cent) the lesion was shown to be a primary or metastatic pulmonary tumour and in 162 patients (18 per cent) the lesion was a chronic inflammation or a pulmonary infarct. The commonest pulmonary lesion judged so closely to mimic pulmonary carcinoma that management by exploratory thoracotomy and diagnostic pulmonary resection was mandatory was pulmonary tuberculosis (in 82 patients); other lesions encountered were cavitated (in eight patients) and non-cavitated (in 61 patients) pneumonias; pulmonary gummata (in two patients); progressive massive fibrosis (in four patients) and a pulmonary infarct (in five patients). It is estimated that in perhaps 60 patients (6·5 per cent of the total) with non-tumorous lesions the pulmonary resection undertaken was needless, or of unnecessary magnitude, and some of these resections might have been avoided if skilled interpretation of frozen sections had constantly been available.

DETAILED and appropriate investigation of the patient who presents with a single peripheral pulmonary opacity—by clinical and radiographic examination; comparison of present films with all previous radiographs; by bronchoscopy and perhaps by thoracoscopy; by the bacteriological and histological examination of sputum; and by a period of observation sufficiently long to allow acute inflammatory lesions to clear and yet sufficiently brief to avoid providing a primary pulmonary tumour with the opportunity of growth to an unmanageable size—is commonly unhelpful and there is then the need to make recourse to exploratory thoracotomy, which provides the opportunity both for diagnosis and treatment. How common is it to resect needlessly, because it is not a carcinoma, a peripheral pulmonary lesion?

In the 15-year period, 1949 to 1963, when 4,000 patients with pulmonary carcinoma were investigated in the regional Thoracic Unit in Edinburgh, pulmonary resection was undertaken in 609 patients—segmental resection in 17, pneumonectomy in 290 and lobectomy in 302—in the knowledge that the appearances at bronchoscopy were normal and in these patients it was later established, by histological examination of the resected specimen, that resection had been undertaken for bronchial carcinoma. In many of these patients the diagnosis of bronchial carcinoma was evident once the chest had been opened. In a further 122 patients exploratory thoracotomy was undertaken with a view to pulmonary resection in the belief that a peripheral lesion was a carcinoma, and resection was either frustrated because of the extent of mediastinal invasion or rendered pointless by the extent of tumour dissemination. Biopsy was made from the primary lesion, in all instances where a planned resection was abandoned, and a lesion not resected in this way was never shown not to be a carcinoma. Thoracotomy was, therefore, undertaken in 731 patients without pre-operative histological confirmation of the diagnosis of bronchial carcinoma other than by the finding of tumour cells in sputum. It became standard practice to search for tumour cells in sputum only after 1955, but during the period when sputum was examined in this way, tumour cells were found in the sputa from only 7 per cent of patients in whom this was the only source of histological information regarding the nature of a pulmonary lesion before operation, and the decision to manage the pulmonary lesion in these patients was made without reference to the finding of tumour cells in the sputum —in fact before histological reports on the examination of sputa were available, because many reports became available only after thoracotomy was undertaken and resection completed. Throughout the period under discussion, it was standard practice to manage by exploratory thoracotomy a persistent peripheral pulmonary shadow in a patient suitable in other respects for an operation, in circumstances which made bronchial carcinoma as the cause of the peripheral shadow a reasonable, if only an alternative, diagnosis, and failure to find tumour cells in the sputum did not, at any time, alter the decision to manage by exploratory thoracotomy a peripheral pulmonary lesion which, on other grounds, was thought to be a tumour.

As a corollary to this attitude towards the management of peripheral pulmonary shadows judged, on reasonable grounds by experts, possibly to indicate bronchial carcinoma, it is necessary to record the number of exploratory thoracotomies and pulmonary resections undertaken in the same period and in the same circumstances for lesions either recognised at exploration or shown by histological examination after resection, not to be bronchial carcinomata.

Pulmonary resection was undertaken in nine patients for lesions shown by histological examination of the resected specimen to be a sarcoma— unqualified in three, lymphosarcoma in two, fibrosarcoma, either primarily pulmonary with parietal invasion, or vice versa, in three, and rhabdomyosarcoma in one. Distinction between carcinoma and sarcoma, for the purpose of patient management, is probably a quibble.

Isolated peripheral pulmonary metastases from extra-thoracic primary tumours were resected in 16 patients, in two sets of circumstances—in patients known to have had a previously managed extra-thoracic primary tumour; and in patients managed as if the pulmonary tumour was a primary, in whom the diagnosis of pulmonary metastases was made after histological examination of the resected specimens, and in whom the silent primary tumour was demonstrated by appropriate investigation after recovery from pulmonary resection. Of the 16 patients, there was an unsuspected silent primary in four, which was renal in two, colonic in one and testicular in one. It was recognised in the remaining 12 patients that the new pulmonary lesion for which investigation was being undertaken might represent a metastasis from a primary extra-thoracic tumour managed six to 17 years earlier. Other metastases were not demonstrated by clinical or special investigation in this group of patients, and the pulmonary lesion was, therefore, resected—by lobectomy in nine patients and by pneumonectomy in three. Metastases—from renal carcinoma in four, from mammary carcinoma in five, from carcinoma of the bladder in two, and from carcinoma of the uterus in one—as the cause of the pulmonary lesion were demonstrated by histological examination of the resected specimens. In the same period a carcinoma unequivocally primary in the lung was resected in three patients previously managed surgically for mammary carcinoma, in four patients previously irradiated for carcinoma of the larynx, in two patients who had had a colectomy for carcinoma, in three patients managed by oesophago-gastrectomy for carcinoma of the gastro-oesophageal junction, in 17 patients previously managed by irradiation or excision for malignant skin tumours, in two patients who had undergone hysterectomy for carcinoma, in a woman who had been irradiated for a skin tumour, managed by mastectomy for mammary carcinoma, and who later died from a gastric tumour, and in a man whose peripheral malignant melanoma had been managed by amputation of the leg. A pulmonary lesion which develops in a patient previously managed for a malignant extra-thoracic tumour is likely, but not certain, to be a pulmonary metastasis. If the pulmonary lesion is not a metastasis, to neglect the opportunity of managing it surgically at an early stage is unfortunate—and in these circumstances lesions are often detected at an early stage because patients in whom a tumour has been dealt with surgically or by irradiation are usually closely followed. If a pulmonary lesion proves to be a metastasis, its resection should not seriously modify prognosis by shortening life if it is one of many metastases, the others not having been recognised; and if it is the only metastasis, long survival may be achieved. Long survival following resection of a metastasis, and possibly even of the primary tumour, is more likely to reflect the natural behaviour of a particular tumour than surgical proficiency. Some patients harbour slowly growing malignant tumours for decades. Lobectomy for metastasis from mammary carcinoma was undertaken in three women, six, nine and 14 years respectively after mastectomy for the primary tumour; in these three patients other metastases became evident four, eight and 11 years respectively after resection of the pulmonary metastasis, when in two of the three patients the exhibition of appropriate hormone therapy was followed by clinical and radiographic restoration to normal; the third patient died within three months with widespread metastases.

In the same period peripheral pulmonary lesions were recognised, without recourse to exploratory thoracotomy, as metastatic in 104 patients who had been managed earlier for a primary extra-thoracic tumour. Recognition of the pulmonary lesion as metastatic was possible because of related lymph glandular metastases; because of multiplicity of the pulmonary lesion; because of related pleural effusion which allowed of the replacement of the effusion with air, thoracoscopy, and biopsy; by biopsy of parietal pleura during management of empyema thoracis by open drainage; or by biopsy of an associated rib lesion. The commonest sites of the original primary tumours were breast (42 patients), kidney (12 patients), colon (nine patients), cervix or body of uterus (eight patients each), prostate and rectum (five patients each); there were one or two examples of pulmonary metastases from previously managed tumours in several other sites. In only three patients in addition to the 104 did pulmonary metastases from an extra-thoracic primary erode a bronchus and become visible at bronchoscopy—that is, present as a central type of tumour from which an informative biopsy could be made at bronchoscopy. While bronchial compression, particularly with intra-thoracic metastases from mammary carcinoma, is not uncommon, the bronchial mucosa is, in these circumstances, usually normal and information of value is rarely obtained from a biopsy made at bronchoscopy.

Also in the same period, 49 other patients with pulmonary metastases were investigated in whom the site of the primary tumour was not found until necropsy, which in 32, demonstrated a small unsuspected primary—in gut, thyroid, pancreas or supra-renal. In this group of 49 patients the lung was only one of many sites of tumour spread, and in all but 11 histological evidence of a malignant tumour was found by examination of biopsy material obtained by lymph gland resection, pleural biopsy at thoracoscopy, or other manoeuvre, but the histological appearances were not sufficiently well differentiated to ascribe the primary tumour to a particular site.

A variety of chronic inflammatory pulmonary lesions may mimic or co-exist with pulmonary carcinoma. Thus, pulmonary carcinoma and active pulmonary tuberculosis are known to have co-existed in 69 patients—one a boy of 19 years—but in some of these patients the tumour was not a surgical proposition. Exploratory thoracotomy was undertaken, in the period under discussion, in 82 patients in all of whom sputum examination before operation had failed to demonstrate the presence of either tumour cells or tubercle bacilli. In all, the pulmonary lesion was peripheral in type, the appearances at bronchoscopy were normal, and plain films (and, in many, tomography) had failed to show evidence such as calcification or satellite shadows which made more likely the diagnosis of pulmonary tuberculosis. In many the diagnosis of carcinoma was favoured because the pulmonary lesion was cavitated, and anti-tuberculous drugs had not yet been exhibited—a combination of circumstances which, had the lesion been tuberculous, made it reasonable to expect a positive sputum. At exploratory thoracotomy in these 82 patients, 62 of whom were men, the lesion was thought most likely to be tuberculous in 45 who were, therefore, submitted only to segmental resection. Lobectomy was undertaken in 26 and pneumonectomy in eight patients, still with the diagnosis of bronchial carcinoma foremost in the mind of the surgeon—all were shown to have pulmonary tuberculosis on histological examination of the resected specimen. In three patients the lesion was found to be an inter-lobar empyema and this was enucleated. Three of the 82 tuberculous lesions managed in the circumstances outlined were resected in 1949, and the number of resections in each subsequent year until 1963 were 4, 3, 4, 6, 4, 9, 9, 9, 7, 6, 6, 5, 2, 5. In 39 of the 82 patients there were available, for comparison with recent films, a chest radiograph made, for whatever purpose, two to six years before presentation to the Thoracic Unit, and one of the reasons for favouring the diagnosis of carcinoma in these patients was the normality of these earlier radiographs. Segmental resection is not an excessive resection for pulmonary tuberculosis in circumstances which make it unacceptable not to undertake exploratory thoracotomy—especially as it has always been the habit to undertake this variety of exploratory operation with a patient under treatment with the three standard anti-tuberculous drugs—chemotherapy starting some days before operation and continuing at least until the histological report on the resected specimen is available. In the same circumstances, lobectomy is also probably not an excessive resection—from the operative notes, if the diagnosis of tuberculosis had been established, segmental resection, rather than lobectomy, might have been undertaken in some of these patients. Pneumonectomy, on the other hand, is an acceptable operation for pulmonary tuberculosis only where the lung is unequivocally destroyed. The eight pneumonectomies were all undertaken at a time when a resection of this extent was virtually standard for pulmonary carcinoma—before 1953—and they were undertaken because the surgeon believed that bronchial carcinoma was the cause of the lesion found at thoracotomy. It is most unlikely that pneumonectomy would ever again be undertaken for a tuberculous lesion, in the circumstances under discussion, in the absence of surgical accident or error during a smaller resection.

Progressive massive fibrosis was commonly recognised in the period under discussion on chest radiographs of miners referred for other purposes; 67 patients were referred specifically for the investigation of a pulmonary lesion thought by referring physicians unlikely to be the consequence of progressive massive fibrosis and most likely to represent a pulmonary carcinoma; in 63 of these patients either additional information was gathered in the Thoracic Unit which made the diagnosis of progressive massive fibrosis reasonably certain and obviated the need for exploratory thoracotomy, or other circumstances precluded exploratory thoracotomy and subsequent progress of the lesion established the diagnosis of progressive massive fibrosis. In four patients recent appearance and the rate of growth of a unilateral pulmonary lesion made the diagnosis of pulmonary carcinoma so likely that lobectomy was undertaken; all survived resection; in all histological examination of the resected specimen established the diagnosis of progressive massive fibrosis; clearly none could afford unnecessarily to lose functioning lung.

In the period under discussion the diagnosis of pulmonary infarction was made in 127 patients referred to the Thoracic Unit for the investigation of haemoptysis, pleural effusion, a pulmonary opacity or a combination of these abnormalities. In five other patients exploratory thoracotomy was undertaken in the belief that the cause of a pulmonary opacity was a peripheral carcinoma; the findings in one were sufficiently suggestive of carcinoma for lobectomy to be undertaken; in four the lesion was thought on exploration so unlikely to be a carcinoma that a segmental resection was made; one of these last mentioned four died from coronary thrombosis on the fourth post-operative day. The histological diagnosis from the resected specimens in these five patients was that of pulmonary infarction.

Two female patients in whom a large peripheral pulmonary lesion was managed by pneumonectomy—one in 1949 and one in 1951—were shown to have had a pulmonary gumma after histological examination of the resected specimens. In neither had appropriate serological examinations been made during investigations to establish the diagnosis of syphilis. One of these patients died at operation from haemorrhage the consequence of damage to the azygos vein.

Of 81 patients managed for acute or chronic lung abscess in the period under discussion, 17 required pulmonary resection; of these 17 patients eight fall into the category of patients submitted to thoracotomy and pulmonary resection because a radiographically cavitated peripheral pulmonary lesion was thought most likely to be a pulmonary carcinoma. All were relatively well; in none was there a history suggestive of acute lung abscess; all are probably better classified as having chronic destructive pneumonia. Lobectomy was undertaken in six of these patients and pneumonectomy in two. Of the eight patients, one died from brain abscess and one from meningitis after a complicated convalescence; one died after a series of events—empyema as a complication of the original lobectomy, broncho-pleural fistula, completion of pneumonectomy as the only way of managing the fistula, and finally death from haemorrhage the consequence of infective disruption of the pulmonary arterial closure; and post-operative empyema complicated recovery in three of the remaining five. A large number of patients—1,083—were referred to the Thoracic Unit in the period under review because a non-cavitated pulmonary lesion failed to show radiographic evidence of clearing in a period of time sufficiently short to make acceptable the diagnosis only of " pneumonia ". Subsequent behaviour in most of these patients made reasonably certain the diagnosis of a non-specific pulmonary infection and complete clearing of the opacity made unlikely the diagnosis of pulmonary carcinoma; all had normal bronchi. Inevitable delay in referral after clinical suspicion had initially been raised rarely made it necessary to reach a decision on management in a patient with a peripheral pulmonary shadow without a series, for comparison, of at least three chest radiographs, made over five to seven weeks; but while progressive and unequivocal diminution in size and density of a pulmonary shadow diminishes the likelihood of the shadow being the consequence of a pulmonary carcinoma, it does not render this diagnosis unacceptable, and continued surveillance of all patients in whom changing pulmonary shadows have been found is necessary. In 61 of the 1,083 patients a pulmonary shadow failed to diminish or was ingravescent; collateral evidence, such as finger clubbing, haemoptysis, loss of weight, and so on, supported the diagnosis of bronchial carcinoma; in this group of patients diagnostic thoracotomy was undertaken, and in all some form of pulmonary resection was completed—pneumonectomy in 12 (all before 1954), lobectomy in 29, segmental resection in 12 and biopsy only in eight. In all, histological examination of the resected specimen showed the lesion to be a non-specific chronic inflammation. Of the 61 patients 55 were men and all smoked. Two men died as the direct consequence of operation—pneumonectomy in one and lobectomy in the other—both from respiratory infection and respiratory insufficiency. Two patients in this group, who had been submitted to lobectomy, later developed pulmonary carcinoma—one in the same lung from which the lobe had been resected and the other in the opposite lung—eight and 10 years after the original operation, respectively. In these two patients the possibility must be recognised that the original lesion for which resection had been undertaken was in fact a carcinoma, that histological material submitted had been misinterpreted, inadequately scrutinised, or had been incomplete; the original specimens are no longer available for scrutiny and slides which remain do not show evidence of tumour; these rare instances justify the preservation of all resected specimens.

From these figures some facts can be extracted. In the period under review exploratory thoracotomy was undertaken in 918 patients because each had been found to have a persistent peripheral pulmonary shadow which, in the opinion of experts, might have been caused by a pulmonary tumour. Of these 918 patients, 756 (82 per cent) were shown to have a pulmonary tumour—bronchial carcinoma in 731, sarcoma in nine, and an isolated pulmonary metastasis from an extra-thoracic primary tumour in 16. The remainder—162 patients (18 per cent)—were shown to have some form of chronic inflammatory lesion or a pulmonary infarct. In this group of 162 patients management at exploratory thoracotomy was by segmental resection, pulmonary biopsy, or the enucleation of an inter-lobar empyema in 72 because the macroscopic features of the lesion made unlikely the diagnosis of pulmonary carcinoma. Lobectomy was undertaken in 66 patients either because the lesion was still thought most likely to be a tumour or because its size precluded a smaller resection. Pneumonectomy was undertaken in 24 patients in the belief that the lesion was a pulmonary tumour. Seven of the 162 patients died in the post-operative period—two after pneumonectomy, four after lobectomy, and one after segmental resection. Half of the patients who were shown not to have a pulmonary tumour were shown to have pulmonary tuberculosis. In this series diagnostic thoracotomy was, in most patients, synonymous with diagnostic pulmonary resection. Diagnostic pulmonary resection ranged from biopsy to pneumonectomy. Diagnostic pneumonectomy was not undertaken after 1954.

Examination of frozen sections was not a part of the routine but was occasionally made available by the accessibility of appropriate pathologists.

It is difficult to define the place of frozen section examination in the management of peripheral pulmonary lesions. If a skilled service is routinely and consistently available, it will obviously be used and some needless resections will be avoided. In this series diagnostic pneumonectomy would probably always have been avoided, but a needless resection of this extent has not been undertaken since 1954—probably for no other reason than the change in attitude towards the extent of resection by which pulmonary carcinoma is adequately managed, lobectomy now being, where possible, preferable to pneumonectomy. Where the diagnosis of pulmonary tuberculosis is made by examination of frozen sections, there can be few surgeons who would not complete the resection of an isolated lesion, the diagnosis of tuberculosis having been established with the chest still open and with the exploration having been undertaken on a patient in receipt of adequate anti-tuberculous chemotherapy. All the segmental resections and some of the lobectomies for tuberculosis in this series would, therefore, have been made despite the availability of an histologist skilled in the interpretation of frozen sections. Some of the lobectomies for tuberculosis would probably have been less extensive resections. It is calculated—at least partly as a guess—that 60 of the 90 resections greater than segmental resection would have been avoided or would have been smaller resections, if an accurate histological diagnosis had been supplied once the thoracotomy had been made. Therefore, of the 918 resections undertaken in patients with peripheral pulmonary shadows, 60 (6·5 per cent) may be regarded as unnecessary resections or resections of an unnecessary magnitude. It is calculated that some of these resections might have been avoided if skilled interpretation of frozen sections had constantly been available. It must, however, always be recognised that a biopsy made at thoracotomy from a large lesion for the purpose of examination of a frozen section may not be representative of the whole lesion, and that, in many instances, biopsy for the purpose of frozen section may well amount to a formal segmental resection or lobectomy. The point which must be clearly established is that diagnostic pneumonectomy is never likely to be a justifiable procedure and, in this series, diagnostic pneumonectomy was not undertaken after 1954.

IX

Management other than Surgical because of Dissemination of Tumour

SUMMARY

Management in 1,834 patients (45·9 per cent) was other than surgical because of metastases or extra-pulmonary extension of tumour.

In 10·6 per cent of the series a cervical node on the same side as the primary tumour was the site of metastasis, and in nearly half of this group the cervical lymph node metastasis was the only evidence of spread of tumour. A cervical lymph-glandular metastasis was the commonest single clinical evidence of dissemination of bronchial carcinoma. Contralateral cervical glandular metastasis from the right lung to the left side of the neck was nearly as common as from the left lung to the right side of the neck. Contralateral and bilateral cervical glandular metastases were each demonstrated in fewer than 2 per cent of patients. Lymphangitis carcinomatosa was seen radiographically in 24 patients.

Presentation in 3·3 per cent of patients was with cerebral metastases, and in 2 per cent of patients osseous metastases constituted the only evidence of tumour spread at the time of first investigation; ribs and vertebrae were the commonest sites of osseous metastases.

In 1·6 per cent of patients there was nodular hepatomegaly and in 1 per cent there were pulmono-pulmonary metastases when first these patients were investigated; this was the only evidence of tumour dissemination in these two groups at that time.

Obstruction of the superior vena cava, present in 4·6 per cent of patients on presentation for investigation, was commonly associated with a tumour in the right upper lobe and with cervical glandular metastases, and occasionally with paralysis of the right vocal cord. The number of women and the number with undifferentiated tumours was higher than in the series as a whole. It was usually possible quickly to relieve the symptoms and signs of caval obstruction by irradiation; recurrence of caval obstruction was common and usually a herald of death.

The other indications of mediastinal invasion demonstrated by investigation—displacement of the barium-filled oesophagus, phrenic palsy and interruption of the left recurrent laryngeal nerve—were present together or separately in nearly 9 per cent of patients. The pulmonary opacity in 132 patients who presented with a left vocal cord palsy as the only evidence of extra-pulmonary extension of tumour was left-sided in all but nine. Survival time from the onset of hoarseness of voice was surprisingly long.

Proximal extension of tumour, seen at bronchoscopy and established by biopsy, precluded surgical management in 4·5 per cent of patients. Adenocarcinoma rarely extended in this way; a disproportionately large number of tumours which extended proximally were right-sided.

In 1 per cent of patients there were cutaneous or subcutaneous metastases as the only evidence of tumour spread at the time of first investigation.

MANAGEMENT in 1,834 patients (45·9 per cent) was other than surgical because of clinical, radiographic, fluoroscopic, bronchoscopic or thoracoscopic evidence of metastasis or extra-pulmonary extension of tumour. To facilitate discussion of this large number of cases they have been grouped in such a way that each of the recognised manifestations of dissemination of bronchial carcinoma can be separately listed, with indication of the number of patients in whom a particular contra-indication to surgical management was the only known evidence of tumour spread, and the number in whom this was one of more indications of dissemination.

I. CERVICAL GLANDULAR METASTASES

Cervical gland biopsy was made in 796 of 4,000 patients with bronchial carcinoma. In 217 patients metastases were not demonstrated in the resected gland; in two of these 217 biopsies the changes of tuberculosis and in five those of sarcoidosis were recognised; in the remainder the gland was either called normal or was said to show non-specific reactive hyperplasia. Cervical gland biopsy was undertaken in all cases because a gland was clinically palpable; scalene node biopsy, in patients without a palpable cervical node, was not undertaken.

In 579 (14·5 per cent of the whole series) of the 796 patients in whom a cervical gland was removed, metastases from bronchial carcinoma were recognised. In 424 (10·6 per cent) patients the metastasis in a cervical node was on the same side as the primary tumour; in 77 patients (1·9 per cent) the cervical node was on that side of the neck opposite to the primary pulmonary tumour; in 78 patients (1·9 per cent) invaded cervical glands were bilateral.

1. Ipsilateral Cervical Glandular Metastases. In 190 of the 424 patients with ipsilateral cervical glandular metastases, the cervical glandular metastasis was the only evidence, on clinical, radiographic, fluoroscopic and bronchoscopic examination, of extension of the tumour outwith the lung; in the remaining 234 patients there was various additional evidence of extra-pulmonary dissemination of tumour. Thus, in 34 patients there was clinical evidence of obstruction of the superior vena cava; in 24 the liver was enlarged and nodular and in another 24 a recurrent laryngeal nerve was interrupted, in all but two the left recurrent laryngeal nerve; 22 patients had osseous metastases and in another 22 displacement of the barium-filled oesophagus was demonstrated; in 19 the bronchoscopic findings precluded surgical management because of involvement of the main carina, the trachea, or both main bronchi; in a further group of 19 there were cerebral metastases, and four of these 19 with cerebral metastases presented with only cerebral symptoms; 17, all with pleural effusion, were shown, by biopsy at thoracoscopy, to have pleural metastases; the primary tumour in 16 was apical and in them the clinical and radiographic features of Pancoast's syndrome were present; a phrenic nerve was paralysed in six and five had pulmono-pulmonary metastases; in four there were cutaneous or subcutaneous metastases and in another four there were radiographic changes interpreted as those of lymphangitis carcinomatosa; in two there was a right supra-hilar shadow, separate from the primary tumour, interpreted as enlargement of the " azygos " gland; in one there was a metastasis in the thyroid gland, in another in a tonsil and in a third in the tongue; in 13 metastases were multiple.

Of the 190 patients in whom an ipsilateral cervical glandular metastasis constituted the only evidence of the spread of tumour, three presented because of hypertrophic pulmonary osteo-arthropathy. Nineteen of the 190 were women, of whom the youngest was 37 years of age, the oldest 72, with four in the fifth decade, six in the sixth, and seven in the seventh decade. Of the 171 men, the youngest were 20 and 29 years respectively, three were in the fourth decade, 29 in the fifth, 64 in the sixth, 60 in the seventh and 13 in the eighth. The tumour and the cervical gland, in these 190 patients, were on the left in 75 (39 per cent), whereas in the total number of 424 patients with an ipsilateral cervical glandular metastasis the tumour and gland were left-sided in 213 (50 per cent)—perhaps because, in the natural course of a left pulmonary tumour, it takes longer for the metastasis to declare itself in the left side of the neck and there is therefore more opportunity for the development of other clinically recognisable evidence of spread.

In patients with ipsilateral cervical glandular metastases from bronchial carcinoma the tumour was visible at bronchoscopy in 55 per cent, whether or not the cervical gland was the only evidence of extra-thoracic dissemination. Approximately a third of those with only a cervical gland as evidence of spread, and approximately half of those with other evidence of spread were not treated in any way, and none survived longer than five months; the remainder were managed by irradiation, and all but one had died within a year of treatment. One—a man of 58 years with a cervical glandular metastasis from an undifferentiated right peripheral tumour—died two years after irradiation.

The tumours in the 190 patients with only an ipsilateral cervical gland were undifferentiated in 60 per cent (called " oat-cell " in an eighth of these) whereas in the group of 234 patients with evidence of spread in addition to an ipsilateral gland the tumour was undifferentiated in only a third. In 32 patients, five of them women, the tumour was an adenocarcinoma and in exactly half of these the cervical lymph-glandular metastasis was the only evidence of spread. The tumours in the rest were squamous, except in six, where there was offered a histological diagnosis which differed for the biopsy made at bronchoscopy from that made in the neck. Thus in two of these six the gland was said to show invasion by undifferentiated carcinoma and the bronchial biopsy invasion by squamous carcinoma; in two the gland showed squamous carcinoma while the bronchial biopsy in the one showed undifferentiated carcinoma and in the other adenocarcinoma; in one a biopsy from squamous carcinoma in the bronchus was associated with an undifferentiated tumour in the neck and in the last an undifferentiated carcinoma in the bronchus metastasised as an adeno-carcinoma to the neck.

Of patients with ipsilateral cervical glandular metastases, with or without other evidence of dissemination of tumour, 14 claimed never to have smoked— eight women, four with squamous tumours, two with undifferentiated tumours

and two with adenocarcinoma; and six men, two with squamous tumours, three
with undifferentiated tumours and one with an adenocarcinoma.

2. Contralateral Cervical Lymph-Glandular Metastases. Of 4,000 patients
with bronchial carcinoma 77 were found, at the time of their first admission
for investigation, to have cervical lymph-glandular metastases on that side of
the neck opposite to the primary pulmonary tumour; in 44 the primary pulmonary tumour was on the left and the cervical metastasis on the right, and in 33
the primary tumour was right-sided with left-sided cervical glandular metastases—experience strikingly different from that related by Nohl,[1] and similar
to that reported by Onuigbo.[2] Of the 77 patients eight were women, of whom
the youngest were 42 and 53 years respectively, and six were in the seventh
decade; one woman of 60 years, with left cervical glandular metastases from
a right lower lobar undifferentiated carcinoma denied ever having smoked. Of
the 69 men, the two youngest were 36 and 38 years, respectively, 11 were in
the fifth decade, 22 in the sixth, 29 in the seventh, four in the eighth, and the
oldest was 90 years—the oldest but one in the whole series.

Of the right-sided pulmonary tumours, seven were in the upper lobe, and
only one of these was associated with a visible bronchoscopic abnormality;
six were in the lower lobe, and three of these were tumours visible at bronchoscopy. In five patients tumour obstructed the lower part of the main bronchus
and was associated with shrinkage of the middle and lower lobes; 11 of the
tumours on the right were called " hilar ", and five of these were associated
with a bronchoscopic abnormality; in four the only radiographic abnormality
on the right was a pleural effusion, and in none of these patients was there a
significant bronchoscopic abnormality. Of the 33 right-sided tumours, therefore, 19 were peripheral and 14 central in type.

Of the left-sided tumours, 12 were in the upper lobe, four of these visible
at bronchoscopy; 10 were in the lower lobe, seven of them visible at bronchoscopy, 10 were described as " hilar ", four of these associated with a
bronchoscopic abnormality; eight were in the left main bronchus, all visible at
bronchoscopy but not all occluding the bronchus; in four patients the only
radiographic abnormality on the left was a pleural effusion, and in none of
these was there an associated bronchoscopic abnormality. Of the 44 left-sided
tumours, therefore, 20 were peripheral and 24 central in type.

Biopsy at bronchoscopy confirmed the diagnosis of bronchial carcinoma
in the 38 patients with central tumours, and in these the histological features
of the biopsy made at bronchoscopy tallied with those of the cervical gland
biopsy.

Of the 77 cervical glands resected, the histological features in 46 were
those of undifferentiated carcinoma, called " oat-cell " in seven; of squamous
carcinoma in 24 and of adenocarcinoma in seven. In 49 patients of this group
of 77 it was possible sooner or later to obtain at necropsy sufficient information
to make it certain that the primary tumour had been allocated to the correct

[1] Nohl, H. C. (1962). *The Spread of Carcinoma of the Bronchus*. London: Lloyd-Luke.
[2] Onuigbo, W. B. (1962). Contra-lateral cervical node metastases in lung cancer. *Thorax*, **17**, 201.

side; in seven of these patients an ipsilateral gland had become clinically recognisable, three to six months after these patients had originally been investigated, and in all shortly before death.

In addition to contralateral cervical glandular metastases, other evidence of widespread dissemination of tumour was adduced in 54 patients. In eight the superior vena cava was obstructed; in 16, one of whom presented with dysphagia, the barium-filled oesophagus was displaced, in five the ipsilateral phrenic nerve interrupted, and in seven phrenic paresis and oesophageal displacement were together demonstrated; in seven the left recurrent laryngeal nerve was interrupted; six had nodular hepatomegaly; osseous metastases were demonstrated in two and in two others subcutaneous lumps were shown histologically to be metastases; the last of this group had diffuse lymphatic infiltration of carcinoma throughout the lung which harboured the primary tumour.

One patient with contralateral cervical glandular metastases presented because of the symptoms of hypertrophic pulmonary osteoarthropathy; one was found incidentally to have a positive sputum with active pulmonary tuberculosis.

Five patients with pleural effusion were managed by the instillation of nitrogen mustard, 43 were managed by irradiation and 34 were not offered any specific therapy. of the 77, 43 had died within six months of admission, 16 others died less than a year after investigation, another 12 within 18 months, and the survival time of six is not known.

3. Bilateral Cervical Lymph-Glandular Metastases. Of 4,000 patients with bronchial carcinoma bilateral cervical lymph-glandular metastases were found in 78, but in only five of these did the cervical lesions constitute the only evidence of extra-pulmonary dissemination of tumour recognisable on standard clinical, radiographic, fluoroscopic and bronchoscopic investigation. Thus, bilateral cervical lymph-glandular metastases were associated, in 15 patients, with obstruction of the superior vena cava; in nine patients there was bronchoscopic evidence of advanced dissemination—tracheal compression, involvement of both main bronchi or an ulcerated and broadened main carina; in eight patients there was radiographic evidence of glandular spread, with unequivocal abnormalities at both hila, or right para-tracheal opacities diagnostic of glandular spread, and in one patient there were pulmono-pulmonary metastases; mediastinal invasion was common, in the form of recurrent laryngeal nerve palsy in eight, phrenic paresis in three and displacement of the barium-filled oesophagus in four, one of whom presented with dysphagia; nodular hepatomegaly was recognised in eight patients, and in two others a mass in the hypochondrium was considered, clinically, to be a supra-renal metastasis, an opinion which was shown at necropsy to be correct; in five patients there were cutaneous or subcutaneous metastases, in three osseous metastases and in one cerebral metastases, while in five patients there was clinical evidence of widespread metastases.

Of those with bilateral cervical glandular metastases the youngest was a man of 39; there were nine women, all in the sixth or seventh decades, in which were also most of the men. One woman, with a right upper lobar undifferentiated carcinoma, denied ever having smoked; all the other patients in this group smoked. The tumour in 50 patients was an undifferentiated carcinoma (called " oat-cell " in four of these), in 25 a squamous carcinoma, and in three an adenocarcinoma. Where radiographic abnormalities were unilateral, right-sided primary tumours were a little more common than left.

In this group of patients death within four weeks of investigation, with the patient never well enough to leave hospital, was common, and few were regarded as suitable for management even by irradiation. There were only three patients who survived longer than six months. A man, 56 years of age at the time of irradiation for a right hilar opacity associated with metastases from undifferentiated carcinoma to glands in both sides of the neck, died with diffuse metastases, three and a half years after irradiation; a woman, 63 at the time of investigation which showed her to have an undifferentiated carcinoma with bilateral cervical glandular metastases and a left recurrent laryngeal nerve palsy, was managed by irradiation and four years later required further irradiation because of tracheal compression with stridor—she died six years after the first investigation; a man of 51 years with bilateral cervical glandular metastases from a carcinoma called " oat-cell ", bilateral hilar shadows, paralysis of the left vocal cord and left phrenic palsy, was managed by irradiation and is alive five years later.

II. OTHER LYMPH-GLANDULAR METASTASES

Glandular metastases were found in the axilla in 12 patients. In two of these the primary pulmonary lesion was on the left and the axillary gland on the right. In the remaining 10 patients the axillary gland and the pulmonary tumour were on the same side. In none of these patients was there clinical or radiographic evidence of direct extension from primary tumour to axilla and in none was there other clinical evidence of glandular metastases. In two patients other than the previously mentioned 12 an axillary gland was invaded but in close relation to a pulmonary tumour which invaded the chest wall and was palpable as a lump in the axilla.

Recorded here, although this case could equally well be mentioned with empyema or bronchiectasis with bronchial carcinoma, are the details of a patient whose chronic empyema discharged intermittently from the age of two years, when first the empyema was drained, to the time when he presented at the age of 51 because of a recent increase in discharge from the sinus. Investigation with a view to definitive management of the empyema included bronchography and he was shown to have shrunken and bronchiectatic middle and lower lobes in relation to the right-sided empyema. A small gland in the right axilla was removed by an enthusiastic registrar and this was reported to contain squamous carcinoma. A biopsy was then made from the sinus and this too showed squamous carcinoma. At this juncture the patient declined further management—he had apparently presented himself on many previous occasions at various hospitals and terminated abruptly attempts at management of his chronic infection. It is not known either what became of the patient or whether

97

the axillary glandular metastasis was from carcinomatous change in a chronic sinus track or from primary bronchial carcinoma. This patient is therefore not included in the total of 4,000.

Metastases in a submandibular lymph-gland in two patients and a parotid lymph-gland in one patient were, in these three, the only evidence of spread. Biopsy in all three patients confirmed that the metastasis was in a lymph-gland in close relation to the salivary gland, and not in the salivary gland.

In 22 patients the only contra-indication to surgical management of bronchial carcinoma was radiographic—the demonstration of a paramediastinal opacity above the right pulmonary hilum in the vicinity of the azygos vein. In 17 of the 22 patients the primary tumour was on the right, and in five it was on the left. In 19 of the 22 patients histological confirmation of the diagnosis of bronchial carcinoma was obtained by biopsy at bronchoscopy and in eight the tumour was squamous and in 11 undifferentiated. In three patients the primary tumour was peripheral in type and histological confirmation of the diagnosis was never obtained. In at least 35 other patients, an " azygos " gland is recorded as having been recognised radiographically as one evidence of tumour spread, but not the only contra-indication to surgical management. Eleven patients with right pulmonary tumours and a radiographic opacity which was accepted pre-operatively as an " azygos " gland were managed by exploratory thoracotomy. In nine of these a pulmonary resection was undertaken and in two the tumour was technically irresectable, but in all 11 patients the lesion responsible for the right supra-hilar paramediastinal opacity was an invaded gland which lay deep to the mediastinal pleura between trachea and superior vena cava, with the azygos vein arching over or below the gland. There was an invaded gland at this site in at least 51 other patients with right-sided pulmonary tumours managed surgically but in whose pre-operative chest radiographs there was not a shadow to which glandular metastases in this site could be related.

Bronchial carcinoma in seven patients, on the right in three of these, was not managed surgically because of unequivocal radiographic evidence of an abnormality of the contralateral pulmonary hilum. In five of the seven patients the tumour was undifferentiated and in two squamous. The contralateral hilar abnormality was in each instance accepted as evidence of lymph-glandular dissemination of tumour, and management was by irradiation; all had died within a year.

III. LYMPHANGITIS CARCINOMATOSA

The radiographic appearances interpreted as those of lymphangitis carcinomatosa were seen in 24 patients with bronchial carcinoma and in seven of these patients these radiographic appearances were the only evidence of dissemination of tumour. In the other 17 patients there was further evidence of tumour spread—obstruction of the superior vena cava, cervical lymph-glandular metastases, involvement of the main carina, or metastases in several sites. In the seven patients in whom the radiographic features of lymphangitis carcinomatosa were the only evidence of tumour spread, the appearances at bronchoscopy were normal and histological confirmation of the diagnosis of bronchial carcinoma was achieved only at necropsy; in all seven instances the tumour was a squamous carcinoma. No patient with the radiographic appearances[1] of diffuse lymphatic permeation of tumour throughout one or both lungs—and the appearances were unilateral in six of the 24 cases—survived longer than 10 weeks from admission to hospital.

In the period under review 12 other patients were investigated because of dyspnoea and the radiographic changes of lymphangitis carcinomatosa. All died during the period of investigation, a few days to three weeks after admission. In five the primary tumour was in the pancreas and in none of these was the site of the primary suspected before death. In two patients the primary tumour was gastric; in one a mammary tumour had been managed surgically and by radiotherapy several years earlier and the diffuse lymphatic permeation was related to mediastinal glandular metastases; in two patients lymphatic permeation of carcinoma throughout the lungs was related to a primary pelvic tumour —uterine in one and ovarian in one: and in two patients the primary tumour was renal.

IV. CEREBRAL METASTASES AS A PRESENTING FEATURE

Of 4,000 patients with bronchial carcinoma 133 (3·3 per cent) presented not because of respiratory symptoms, but to medical out-patient, casualty or neurosurgical departments with symptoms and signs of intra-cranial lesions and who, in the course of general investigation in most, but after craniotomy in 11, were shown to have intra-cranial metastases from bronchial carcinoma. Some admitted respiratory symptoms—five had had haemoptysis, four believed themselves to have become breathless, and 11 claimed to have had chest pain— but none had thought it necessary to seek advice for respiratory symptoms. All those with haemoptysis were shown to have bronchoscopically visible tumours; in none with pain was there evidence of chest wall invasion; in none with dyspnoea was the primary pulmonary tumour of a size which, from space occupation alone, could be held to account for dyspnoea.

The commonest neurological disturbance leading to admission to hospital was hemiplegia (21 patients); the recent onset of epilepsy prompted referral for advice in 19, in five of whom epilepsy was Jacksonian in type; personality change, or confusional states in 18 patients, speech defects (dysphasia or aphasia) in 15, and cerebellar disturbances in another 15 precipitated admission; 14 patients were investigated for headache alone, and 10 others for headache with vomiting and visual disturbances; four were admitted in coma from increased intra-cranial tension; 10 were monoparetic and seven presented with an isolated cranial nerve palsy.

Of the 133 patients 12 were women of whom the youngest were 46 and 48 years respectively, and of whom six were in the sixth decade and four in the

[1] Trapnell, D. H. (1964). The radiological appearances of lymphangitis carcinomatosa. *Thorax*, **19**, 251.

seventh decade. Of the 121 men the youngest were 32 and 37 years respectively, 14 were in the fifth decade, 56 in the sixth, 40 in the seventh and nine in the eighth decade.

A histological diagnosis was achieved by biopsy at bronchoscopy in 58 patients; in 75 with peripheral tumours histological confirmation of the diagnosis was achieved in all but 16—by cervical gland biopsy in five (from ipsilateral cervical glands in four and from bilateral cervical gland in one), by aspiration biopsy in three, by craniotomy in 11, and at necropsy in 40. The tumour was called undifferentiated in 63 ("oat-cell" in 12), and squamous in 45, and in nine the tumour was an adenocarcinoma. Right and left tumours were equally common.

The duration of cerebral symptoms before admission was usually less than a month, in some less than a week, and in those patients whose only complaint was headache symptoms had persisted in all for more than three months and in one for 18 months. One patient, with cerebral symptoms for three weeks, had for two years had haemoptysis, for which he had never sought advice.

All patients in this group of 133 died within six months of investigation, and 59 died within a month of admission to hospital.

In seven patients, outwith the group of 133, craniotomy was undertaken to establish the cause of a space-occupying intra-cranial lesion, a tumour was excised, it was believed completely, and the tumour was subsequently shown to be a metastasis from pulmonary carcinoma. In all these patients it was recognised before craniotomy that there was an intra-pulmonary radiographic abnormality which was probably a carcinoma, thoracic surgical advice had been enlisted before craniotomy and the likelihood of the diagnosis of pulmonary carcinoma confirmed, and a plan of action beginning with craniotomy agreed upon. Only four of these patients were subsequently well enough for the second stage of the planned procedure—thoracotomy; pneumonectomy was undertaken in one and lobectomy in three; mediastinal glands were invaded in two; evidence of further cerebral metastases developed in all but one within a year; one is alive five years after completion of surgical management.

In 42 patients, outwith the group of 133, preliminary investigation had not established the presence of cerebral metastases but some aspect of the patient's history or behaviour prompted the record being made that intra-cranial metastases might be present. In this group pulmonary resection was undertaken because it could not be established, by experts, that there were in fact intra-cranial metastases, and investigation included cerebral angiography in 12, lumbar puncture in all, and electro-encephalography in all but one. Within six months of operation it was abundantly clear in all these patients that intra-cranial metastases were increasing in size, and in four the futility of pulmonary resection was clear even before discharge from hospital, because of the unmistakable advance of a cerebral lesion.

There was clinical evidence of cerebral metastases in 31 other patients. None of these presented because of the clinical features associated with cerebral metastases, and in some evidence of cerebral metastases was recognised clinically not at the time of first examination but only later during the period of initial investigation. Admission was, in this group of 31 patients, prompted either because of respiratory symptoms or because of other evidence of spread of tumour such as pain from osseous metastases. Of the 31 patients, 15 had ipsilateral lymph-glandular metastases, three pulmono-pulmonary metastases, and 13 had other evidence of tumour dissemination to bone in three, to liver in three, to skin or subcutaneous tissues in four, and to the mediastinal structures, with oesophageal displacement, phrenic paresis, vocal cord paresis, or a combination of these in three.

V. OSSEOUS METASTASES

In 87 patients osseous metastases constituted the only evidence at the time of first investigation of dissemination of tumour. Ten of these 87 patients were women, of whom the youngest was 34 and the oldest 75; seven were in the seventh or eighth decade. Two women—of 61 and 75 years respectively— denied ever having smoked; in one of these the pulmonary tumour was peripheral and histological confirmation of the diagnosis was not obtained; in the other the tumour was undifferentiated. Of the men, the two youngest were both 38 years of age, eight were in the fifth decade, 17 in the sixth, 43 in the seventh, and seven in the eighth decade.

Of the 87 patients 63 presented because of osteocopic pain. The others presented with respiratory symptoms of which chest pain was one feature.

The commonest site of osseous metastases was the ribs. In 35 patients there were rib metastases—clearly metastases, as opposed to the result of direct costal invasion by the primary pulmonary tumour. In 29 patients the rib metastasis recognised was single, and in six multiple. Six patients presented because of pain of acute onset in relation to coughing, and there was seen radiographically a fracture through a rib metastasis.

The next most common site of osseous metastases from bronchial carcinoma was the vertebrae—in 31 patients. Two of these patients presented because of paraplegia and one because of urinary retention. In three patients the metastases were in the cervical vertebrae, in 10 in the thoracic vertebrae and in eighteen in the lumbar vertebrae.

In six patients osseous metastases were in the femur, in the mid-shaft in one and at the proximal end of the shaft in five. Two of these patients fractured a femur while in the ward being investigated for respiratory symptoms, and the fracture was recognised to be through a metastasis; in these two osseous metastases had not been suspected before the fracture. Pelvic osseous metastases alone were present in five patients—two in the iliac crest, in an ischium in two, and multiple in one. There were single examples of metastasis to a humerus, a clavicle, an acetabulum and the sacrum. The first two of these four were associated with pathological fracture, which was the presenting complaint.

Multiple osseous metastases were present in the remaining six patients— in ribs and both femora in one; ribs and a clavicle in one; vertebrae and pelvis in two; ribs and the sternum in one; and ribs and vertebrae in the last.

Histological confirmation of the diagnosis of bronchial carcinoma was achieved in all but 22 of these patients—at bronchoscopy in 38 and by biopsy from rib, clavicle or sternum in 27. In 39 the tumour was squamous and in 26 undifferentiated.

Of the 87 patients most were irradiated, treatment being directed to the site of osseous metastases in an attempt, in most successful, to relieve pain; all had died within a year of investigation and most had died within six months.

Osseous metastases were found in 48 other patients who had evidence of extra-pulmonary dissemination of tumour in addition to osseous metastases—pulmono-pulmonary metastases in two, cervical glandular metastases in 27 and involvement of several sites in 19. In only one patient, with cervical glandular metastases, is the primary pulmonary tumour known to have been an adenocarcinoma.

VI. HEPATIC METASTASES AS THE ONLY CONTRA-INDICATION TO SURGICAL MANAGEMENT

Of 4,000 patients with bronchial carcinoma 66 had, at the time of presentation for a surgical opinion, nodular hepatomegaly as the only clinical evidence of dissemination of tumour. Of the 66 patients, seven were women and 59 men; the youngest woman was 52 and the oldest 80 years; the youngest man was 38, four men were in the fifth decade, 21 in the sixth, 28 in the seventh, and five were over 70 years, the oldest being 75. Two men presented because of a radiological abnormality detected at routine mass miniature radiography; the others all presented with symptoms, either respiratory or referable to hepatic metastases, or both. Four were jaundiced at the time of first admission; one of the patients with jaundice also had ascites, and four others not recognised as icteric also had ascites.

Histological confirmation of the diagnosis was achieved in 63 of the 66 patients. In 40 the tumour was called undifferentiated, in nine of these " oat-celled ", and in 23 the tumour was squamous in type. Bronchoscopic biopsy permitted histological examination in 43 with central tumours. In 23 with peripheral tumours, in whom the appearances at bronchoscopy were normal, a histological diagnosis was achieved in 20—in 12 at necropsy, in four at limited laparotomy with hepatic biopsy, and in four by gland biopsy some weeks after they first presented, a cervical node having enlarged in the interim. Other evidence of tumour dissemination which developed between first admission and death in this group of patients was personality change suggestive of cerebral metastases in two, vertebral metastases in two, malignant pleural effusion in three, obstruction of the superior vena cava in three, hoarseness of voice in three, and pathological fracture of the humerus in one.

Eighteen of the 66 patients were never well enough to leave hospital—in them, in fact, admission was substantially for terminal care, although none had previously been investigated, either in the Thoracic Unit or elsewhere. All but one were dead within six months of first being investigated; one patient survived for seven months.

Hepatic metastases were common in patients who had other evidence of tumour dissemination. Thus, in four who had the clinical features of superior vena caval obstruction, in 38 with cervical glandular metastases, ipsilateral, contralateral or bilateral, and 21 who had metastases in several sites there were also hepatic metastases.

VII. PULMONO-PULMONARY METASTASES

Of 4,000 patients with bronchial carcinoma 42 were found, when they first presented for investigation, to have radiographic evidence of pulmono-pulmonary metastases as the only evidence of spread of tumour. Of these 42, five were women—the youngest 43 years, the oldest 70, and three in the sixth decade. The two youngest men were 37 and 39 years, respectively, eight were in the sixth decade, 23 in the seventh, and four were over 70 years, the oldest being 80. A woman of 70 years with a squamous carcinoma visible at broncho-scopy in the middle bronchus, and a man of 72 years with an adenocarcinoma visible at bronchoscopy in the right anterior basal bronchus both denied ever having smoked; two men were pipe-smokers; one man had not smoked for 10 years; the smoking habits of five are not recorded; all the others smoked cigarettes.

The histological pattern of the tumour is known in 34 of the 42 patients. Squamous tumours in 15 patients, undifferentiated tumours in four and adeno-carcinomata in three patients were visible at bronchoscopy; cervical lymph-glandular metastases from four peripheral squamous and two undifferentiated tumours developed later and were proven histologically; in two patients submitted to pulmonary biopsy the tumours were squamous; in four patients in whom the histological features of the tumour were unknown before death, necropsy allowed of the making of the diagnosis of squamous carcinoma in two and undifferentiated carcinoma in the other two. Nearly three in every four of the tumours the histology of which is known were shown, therefore, to be squamous in type.

Radiographically pulmono-pulmonary metastases in the 42 patients could be classified as diffuse and bilateral, rarely miliary but equally rarely of a nodule diameter greater than 0·5 mm., in 13 cases; an isolated, often large metastasis in 11; and sparse metastases, 1-4 cm. in diameter, in 18, bilateral in five of these. Where metastases were unilateral, they were ipsilateral in only five instances, and contralateral in 19.

In addition to pulmono-pulmonary metastases, bronchial carcinoma in three patients was associated with cerebral metastases; in six patients with cervical glandular metastases, bilateral in one of these; with diffuse rib metastases in one and vertebral metastases in another; interruption of the left recurrent laryngeal nerve in four and phrenic palsy in two; and displacement of the barium-filled oesophagus in three, one of whom presented with dysphagia.

Presentation, other than in the patient with dysphagia, was a little unusual in only two other patients, both of whom tolerated daily haemoptysis for more than a year before they sought advice.

In two patients the diagnosis of pulmono-pulmonary metastases presented difficulty. Both were coal miners with the radiographic changes of pneumoconiosis; one also had rheumatoid arthritis and in him additional pulmonary shadows were interpreted for some years as those of Caplan's syndrome. Increase in some of the diffusely scattered opacities in the miner without rheumatoid arthritis, and ingravescent dyspnoea, prompted pulmonary biopsy; diminution and then increase in size of some of the shadows interpreted as suggestive of Caplan's syndrome in the other miner prompted a similar course; in both, diffuse pulmonary lesions were palpated at exploratory thoracotomy, and several biopsies in each case demonstrated the presence of diffuse pulmonary metastases of squamous carcinoma. The natural course of the disease in both instances allowed of necropsy, and in neither was there a source of squamous carcinoma outwith the lungs.

In this group of 42 patients, none survived longer than nine months and all but one died within six months of the time of admission to hospital; 11 were never well enough to leave hospital.

VIII. OBSTRUCTION OF THE SUPERIOR VENA CAVA

Of 4,000 patients with bronchial carcinoma 183 (4·6 per cent) had, at the time of first presentation the clinical features of obstruction of the superior vena cava—an incidence very much lower than that reported from The Brompton Hospital[1] where 107 of 732 cases (14 per cent) presented with obstruction of the superior vena cava. From this figure of 183 are excluded two patients who also had Pancoast's syndrome, and a small group of patients who, at the time of first presentation, were shown to have, or suspected of having, pulmonary carcinoma but who declined treatment, and who returned, in two instances two years later, with the clinical features of superior vena caval obstruction and who were then managed by irradiation. Also excluded are those in whom pulmonary carcinoma was originally managed by resection and in whom superior vena caval obstruction developed sooner or later in the postoperative period as evidence of tumour recurrence. Sixty-seven patients are known to have been afflicted in this way, but the incidence of obstruction of the superior vena cava in close relationship to death may have been higher.

Of the 183 patients 26 (14 per cent) were women, of whom the youngest were 29 and 35 years respectively. Seven women were in the fifth decade, eight in the sixth, six in the seventh, and three were 70 years or over, the oldest being 75. The youngest of the 157 men with superior caval obstruction was 25 years, and six others were younger than 40; 23 were in the fifth decade, 60 in the sixth, 55 in the seventh and 12 were older than 70 years, the oldest being 75 years. Of all the patients with superior vena caval obstruction 58 per cent were younger than 60 years, in comparison with 49 per cent in the whole series of 4,000.

[1] Szur, L. & Bromley, L. C. (1956). Obstruction of the superior vena cava in carcinoma of the bronchus. *Br. med. J.*, **2**, 1273.

Six patients in the group claimed never to have smoked—five women, one of them the youngest in the group, and one man. In all six the histological features of the tumour are known—five were squamous and one undifferentiated. The smoking habits of 56 patients in the group of 183 are not known—the highest level of ignorance regarding smoking habits in the whole series. There seems no reasonable explanation for this high level of failure in note-taking, unless it is that so many of these patients were, and all of them looked, so gravely ill, that anamnesis tended to be cursory.

Histological confirmation of the diagnosis of bronchial carcinoma was obtained in 163 of the 183 patients with superior vena caval obstruction—by biopsy from an ipsilateral cervical gland in 34 patients, in 13 of whom a positive biopsy was also obtained at bronchoscopy; by biopsy from a contralateral cervical gland in eight patients, in two of whom a positive biopsy was also obtained at bronchoscopy; biopsy from one of bilateral cervical glands in 15 patients, in five of whom a positive biopsy was also obtained at bronchoscopy; by biopsy at bronchoscopy as the only source of material for histological examination in 89 patients, in 18 of whom the tumour encroached on the trachea, distal to which vision was precluded (in 12 of these the trachea was described as scabbard-shaped) and in 15 of whom the main carina was broad and ulcerated; by formal thoracotomy with mediastinal biopsy in two patients—a girl of 29 years, so as to exclude lymphoma as the cause of caval obstruction, and a man of 60 years with symptoms of obstruction of the superior vena cava for three years, to exclude mediastinal fibrosis as the cause—both of whom had squamous tumours; by the aspiration of a pleural effusion, its replacement with air and visual examination of the pleural surfaces at thoracoscopy, with biopsy, in three patients; and at necropsy in 12 patients in whom histological proof of the diagnosis of pulmonary carcinoma had not been obtained before death.

In 20 patients histological proof of the diagnosis of bronchial carcinoma was never obtained. Of these 20 patients all except two were over 65 years, all were managed by irradiation, and all are known to have died within a year of irradiation. All had pulmonary as well as mediastinal shadows, and it is unlikely that these patients had lymphomata and not pulmonary carcinomata. From the group of 183 patients with superior vena caval obstruction have been deliberately excluded patients in whom histological proof of the diagnosis of carcinoma was not obtained and who may, on other evidence, conceivably have had a lymphoma—and three young people in particular were excluded on this ground. Much of the histological material is still available from the 163 cases in whom histological proof was obtained, and this has been reviewed without the need to alter the opinion originally given—that these tumours were carcinomata. Notwithstanding a deliberate attempt at limiting the number of patients in this group, to avoid including any patient with a lymphoma, the number of women in the group is higher than in the series as a whole, and the number of patients younger than 60 years is also higher.

The histological diagnosis by biopsy in the 163 patients in whom the diagnosis of carcinoma was confirmed was undifferentiated in 99, in 12 of whom the terminology " oat-cell carcinoma " was used, squamous in 63, and adenocarcinoma in only one. The proportion of undifferentiated to squamous tumours is unusually high, when compared with the series as a whole.

Evidence of extra-pulmonary dissemination of tumour other than superior vena caval obstruction was common in this group of patients. At fluoroscopy displacement of the barium-filled oesophagus was demonstrated in 31 patients, seven of whom complained of dysphagia at the time of admission; in 33 other patients phrenic paresis was demonstrated; in a third group, of 12, both oesophageal displacement and phrenic paresis were shown; and in a fourth group, of six patients, phrenic paresis, oesophageal displacement and interruption of the left recurrent laryngeal nerve were demonstrated. In 11 patients recurrent laryngeal nerve palsy was the only indication of mediastinal invasion other than caval obstruction, and in five of the 11 the cord palsy was right-sided. In only one patient with a right cord palsy was there clinically palpable a mass of glands in the right side of the neck, and it must be assumed in the others that the right recurrent laryngeal nerve was interrupted in its course around the subclavian artery at a level which precluded palpation from the neck. Nodular hepatomegaly was recognised in four patients, and diffuse lymphatic permeation of carcinoma throughout both lungs in two others. In one patient a right upper lobar tumour was associated with obstructive emphysema of the middle and lower lobes—a radiographic finding surprisingly rare throughout the series.

Most of the patients in this group of 183 presented within three months of the development of superior vena caval obstruction and many within a month, but 18 tolerated obstructive symptoms for six months or longer, and in one patient, previously mentioned, symptoms had persisted for three years.

Of the 183 patients with superior vena caval obstruction seven died in hospital within three weeks of admission without any form of treatment, and death in these was attributed to progress of disease. Seventeen other patients were considered too ill even for radiotherapy, and all had died within six weeks of admission. The other 159 patients were managed by irradiation. Of these, 100 died within six months of treatment and a further 29 within a year of treatment; 10 patients cannot now be traced, but all were ill at the time of irradiation and have probably died, and probably within a year of treatment. Seventeen patients survived irradiation for more than a year; 11 of these had died within two years, five with recurrence of caval obstruction. Two patients lived for more than two years but less than three years after irradiation; three survived almost exactly three years and one five years, all to die with recurrence of caval obstruction.

Only three patients are known to be alive, two 24 and 26 months respectively following irradiation, and one 10 years following irradiation. This last-mentioned man was 55 at the time of irradiation with an undifferentiated tumour visible in the right upper bronchus, and is entirely well with a normal-looking right upper bronchus at the present time. Expert histologists state categorically that the tumour in this patient was not a lymphoma.

Radiotherapy relieved the clinical features of superior vena caval obstruction in nearly all patients; records show only five patients not to have been relieved of symptoms and signs, but on this score the records are not always explicit; recurrence of the clinical features of obstruction of the superior vena cava was common, two months to as long as five years after irradiation, and was usually a herald of death; irradiation for the second time was often impossible because the permissible dosage had already been administered, and when radiotherapy was repeated, it was less often successful in relieving the obstructive features of the syndrome.

As far as could be judged radiographically, the pulmonary tumour was primarily on the right in most of the 183 patients, and in most of the right tumours the primary was in the right upper lobe. The radiographic abnormality was only on the left in 11 patients—in one the lingular segment was shrunken and opaque, in one the left lower lobe, in two the left upper lobe, in four the left shadow was described as hilar, without pulmonary shrinkage, in two as supra-hilar, and in the last the left hemithorax was uniformly opaque and there was a large left effusion. Bilateral hilar shadows were recognised in five patients, in each with a right supra-hilar extension, and the primary lesion in these patients might have been on either side; in two patients with lymphangitis carcinomatosa the primary site of tumour was uncertain even at necropsy, but was not extra-pulmonary. In all other instances the primary tumour was on the right, and in the right upper lobe in 107—either peripherally and sometimes cavitated in the upper lobe, without lobar shrinkage, or centrally, visible bronchoscopically, and associated with lobar shrinkage and airlessness. A small right effusion was a common radiographic finding; a large effusion was found in eight patients. Right lobar shrinkage other than upper was rare—the right lower lobe was shrunken in four patients, and the middle and lower lobes together in three; the right anterior segment was the only part of the upper lobe to be shrunken and opaque in six patients. Five patients are described as having a broad mediastinum, without more accurate indication regarding the site of the primary lesion.

In addition to the 183 patients discussed above, one patient presented with the clinical features of obstruction of the inferior vena cava; he died within a few days of admission and was shown at necropsy to have intra-pericardial extension of a right hilar tumour, with the intra-pericardial course of the inferior vena cava through a mass of strangulating tumour.

IX. OESOPHAGEAL DISPLACEMENT

Displacement of the barium-filled oesophagus, recognised at fluoroscopy and recorded radiographically, was the only evidence of tumour extension beyond the lung in 138 patients. It was recognised that the interpretation of this finding as evidence of invasion of mediastinal glands by neoplasm was no more than a reasonable guess, that inflammatory lymph-glandular enlargement

107

could equally well be responsible for oesophageal displacement, and that infection distal to central tumours was a possible source of infection from which mediastinal glands might enlarge. However, oesophageal displacement was so common a concomitant of other evidence of tumour spread, such as ulceration of the main carina, involvement by tumour of both main bronchi or of the trachea, phrenic and recurrent laryngeal nerve palsies, and cervical lymph-glandular metastases, that it seemed reasonable to accept oesophageal displacement alone as equally good evidence of lymph-glandular metastases. The recognition of oesophageal displacement at fluoroscopy requires, as does the recognition of all radioscopic and radiographic abnormalities, practice and devoted attention, and the displaced oesophagus must be shown on appropriate films before the abnormality is acceptable. The oesophagus indented by the left main bronchus or the aorta, or displaced in common with the mediastinum or following an unfolded aorta is often interpreted as pathologically displaced by the fluoroscopist.

Of the 138 patients 18 were women, of whom the youngest was 33, six were in the fifth decade, two in the sixth, seven in the seventh and two in the eighth. Two women, both in the seventh decade, one with a squamous and one with an undifferentiated tumour, claimed never to have smoked. A man of 54 with a squamous tumour claimed also never to have smoked. Of the 120 men in this group the youngest was 25 years, seven were in the fourth decade, 16 in the fifth, 42 in each of the sixth and seventh, and 10 in the eighth decade; the oldest were 80 and 83 years respectively. In 49 patients the tumour was a squamous carcinoma and in 70 an undifferentiated carcinoma, called " oat-cell " in 11 of these; in one the tumour was an adenocarcinoma and in one other an alveolar-cell carcinoma; in 17 the tumour was peripheral in type, without a bronchoscopic abnormality, and in these histological confirmation of the diagnosis was not achieved at the time of irradiation; in seven of the 17 necropsy four to 17 months after irradiation supplied a histological diagnosis, of undifferentiated carcinoma in four and of squamous carcinoma in three. In 84 patients the primary tumour was right-sided and in 54 left-sided. Two patients presented because of hypertrophic pulmonary osteo-arthropathy and two with an abnormality on a chest radiograph made for an unrelated purpose and without respiratory symptoms.

Of the 138 patients in whom resection was not suggested as the form of treatment because of oesophageal displacement, 40 had died within six months of investigation, 31 of these after irradiation; 56 others had died within 12 months of investigation, 50 of these after irradiation; 14 others had died within 18 months of irradiation, five within two years, and three died during the third year after irradiation; the remaining 20 are known to have died, all probably within three years, but precise dates of death cannot be found.

Displacement of the barium-filled oesophagus was demonstrated in 31 patients who had, as additional evidence of tumour spread, obstruction of the superior vena cava; in 42 patients who had cervical lymph-glandular metastases; in 59 patients in whom there was evidence at bronchoscopy of unsuitability for surgical management; and in 36 patients who had several contra-indications to surgical management.

Where dysphagia is related to malignant disease the tumour responsible for dysphagia is nearly always in the proximal part of the alimentary tract; the only other common causes of malignant dysphagia are mediastinal metastases from primary pulmonary and primary mammary tumours. Of 4,000 patients with bronchial carcinoma dysphagia was the only presenting complaint in 13, and in 47 other patients dysphagia was one of the presenting complaints. In 30 of these 60 patients oesophageal displacement and compression, demonstrated at fluoroscopy and confirmed at oesophagoscopy, was the only evidence of tumour spread outwith the lung; in none of this group of 30 was the oesophageal mucosa disrupted and in none was there any reasonable doubt that the primary tumour was pulmonary. In the remaining 30 patients there was evidence of tumour spread other than to the mediastinal glands which were responsible for dysphagia, and in these patients there was again no reasonable doubt that the tumour was primarily of the lung. It is not known how many patients developed dysphagia as a terminal event; the number is likely to be considerably higher than the 39 who, whether after a resection for pulmonary carcinoma or after irradiation for pulmonary carcinoma unsuitable for surgical management but without dysphagia at that time, developed dysphagia at a later date, often within a year of treatment. Excluded from the group of 4,000 patients are seven who presented during the period under discussion with dysphagia; in these there was a hilar shadow and squamous carcinoma in the trachea or at the main carina, and in the oesophagus, and four had or later developed a tracheo-oesophageal fistula. These are excluded because it is not known whether the primary tumour in these patients was oesophageal or pulmonary.

Exploratory thoracotomy was undertaken in 30 patients in the knowledge that the barium-filled oesophagus was displaced—in 20 as part of a continuous series in a deliberate attempt to demonstrate the validity of the contra-indication, and in 10 patients, scattered throughout the series, because of doubt regarding the validity of the fluoroscopic interpretation or for reasons which can only be described as emotional.

In the continuous series of 20 patients, managed during a single year, resection was frustrated in 17 because of mediastinal invasion. The oesophagus in the other three in this group was unequivocally displaced by tumorous glands which could be enucleated. In the non-sequential group of 10 patients resection was frustrated in six and completed in four, in one of whom mediastinal glands were not invaded.

X. PHRENIC PARESIS AS THE ONLY CONTRA-INDICATION

Of 4,000 patients with bronchial carcinoma phrenic paresis was the only evidence of extension of tumour outwith the lung in 65, seven of whom were women. The total of 65 patients does not include any patient mentioned elsewhere in the series. None of this group of 65 was managed by thoracotomy.

Of the seven women, the youngest was a girl of 16 years, the oldest was 73, and five were in the sixth decade. The 16-year-old girl, who is also the youngest patient in the whole series, did not smoke, and was shown at bronchoscopy to have a tumour which obstructed the left main bronchus and was associated with paresis of the left phrenic nerve. The tumour was undifferentiated in type, and management was by irradiation; she died six months after treatment had stopped. Of the 58 men, the youngest was 34, eight were in the fifth decade, 21 in each of the sixth and seventh decades, and seven in the eighth decade.

In 49 patients the tumour was visible at bronchoscopy and in these histological confirmation of the diagnosis was obtained by biopsy; in seven other patients a histological diagnosis was achieved only at necropsy, after irradiation in five of these; in nine patients the diagnosis of carcinoma was presumptive; on the ground of an extending pulmonary opacity of peripheral type, with ipsilateral phrenic paresis; in two of the last-mentioned nine, cells in the sputum were said to be suspicious of tumour cells. In 35 patients the tumour was called undifferentiated and in 21 squamous; the phrenic paresis was ipsilateral in all instances, left-sided in 39. The tumours were upper lobar or hilar in 46 patients, and in the remainder in a lower lobe or the middle lobe; in six there was an associated pleural effusion, but in none was this of a size which made difficult the identification of the diaphragmatic dome at fluoroscopy.

Of the 65 patients in this group eight were not treated in any way—because of age, frailty, lack of symptoms, or disinclination on the part of the patient. All had died within a year. The others were all managed by irradiation, and 12 of these were alive at the end of one year. Of the 12, nine died within two years of irradiation, one died three years after irradiation, and two are alive, one nine and one 12 years after irradiation. The nine-year survivor, a man of 55, had a squamous tumour which obstructed the lower part of the right main bronchus and was associated with shrinkage of the middle and lower lobes; he is now overweight, dyspnoeic and still with a right phrenic palsy. The 12-year survivor, a woman of 50 years, had an undifferentiated tumour which obstructed the left lower bronchus. In her case the left dome of the diaphragm now moves normally both with quiet respiration and with sniffing. In both these patients the appearances at bronchoscopy are now normal.

Thoracotomy was undertaken for the management of bronchial carcinoma in 17 patients who had been shown by routine pre-operative investigation to have phrenic paresis. In all these instances the argument proffered for this departure from routine was that the tumour lay adjacent to the pericardium in a lower lobe, and that it might be possible to resect the tumour with part of what was calculated to be a directly invaded pericardium. A resection was completed in 12 patients, and in five patients mediastinal invasion precluded resection. In three patients the phrenic nerve was found not to be invaded, and was shown by direct stimulation not to conduct.

Phrenic paresis was found in two patients who presented because of an abnormality found at mass radiography and who did not have respiratory symptoms; in three patients who presented with hypertrophic pulmonary osteoarthropathy; in two patients with Pancoast's syndrome; in two with pulmono-pulmonary metastases; in three with obstruction of the superior vena cava; and in 14 with cervical lymph-glandular metastases, ipsilateral in six, contralateral in five and bilateral in three. In 18 patients phrenic paresis was associated with metastases in several sites.

Nineteen patients, all men in the sixth, seventh or eighth decade, were shown to have both oesophageal displacement and interruption of a phrenic nerve as the only evidence of extension of tumour outwith the lung. In two the tumour was peripheral in type and histological confirmation of the diagnosis of pulmonary carcinoma was not obtained; in 17 the tumour was central, and of these the tumour was squamous in 10 and undifferentiated in 7 (" oat-cell " in two of these). Two of the 19 were considered too ill for any form of treatment, and of the 17 managed by irradiation 12 had died within six months of treatment and all within a year.

Oesophageal displacement and phrenic paresis were found together in two patients who presented from a mass radiography unit and without respiratory symptoms; in 38 patients with superior vena caval obstruction and in seven with contralateral cervical lymph-glandular metastases. In 25 patients oesophageal displacement and phrenic paresis together were but two of a group of features indicating metastasis or extension of tumour.

XI. LEFT RECURRENT LARYNGEAL NERVE PALSY

Of 4,000 patients with bronchial carcinoma interruption of the left recurrent laryngeal nerve was the only evidence of extra-pulmonary extension of tumour in 132. Hoarseness of voice was the reason for seeking medical advice in 49 of these 132 patients, and in them this symptom was of a duration which varied from three years to two weeks, and in most the complaint was of at least three or four months' duration. In the remaining 83 patients hoarseness of voice was only one of several complaints, which included haemoptysis, dyspnoea and so on, and in some instances the patient did not realise that there was a change in voice. For example, one patient was a postman who thought he was making a slow recovery from an influenzal illness and in him voice change was recognised by an Ear, Nose and Throat surgeon to whom he routinely delivered mail. The youngest patients in this group were a woman of 33 and a man of 39. There were seven women, most in the seventh decade, and two, one with a squamous tumour, who did not smoke. Of the men 14 were in the fifth decade, 48 in the sixth, 40 in the seventh, and 22 in the eighth decade. Five men were pipe smokers, the smoking habits of 12 are not known, and the others smoked cigarettes, 17 of them more than 50 a day.

In this group of 132 patients the left cord was seen at bronchoscopy to be immobile and to lie in the cadaveric position. The related pulmonary opacity was left-sided in all but nine of the 132. The tumour was visible at bronchoscopy in only 47, in 26 of whom the histological features were those of squamous carcinoma, in 19 of an undifferentiated tumour (" oat-cell " in three) and in

111

two of adenocarcinoma. Of the left-sided tumours two-thirds were in the left upper lobe or at the left pulmonary hilum; in many gross shrinkage of the left upper lobe precluded biopsy at bronchoscopy from a tumour visible with an angled telescope. Histological confirmation of the diagnosis of carcinoma was achieved in only a third of the patients in this group at the time of their first investigation, but ultimate histological proof was obtained—by cervical gland biopsy in seven patients nine to 14 months after first investigation, and at necropsy in 23 —in another 30 patients, in 23 of whom the tumour was squamous.

Management in this group of 132 patients was determined by age and symptoms other than hoarseness of voice, because it was argued that irradiation would not restore normal voice, and that, since there was already evidence of mediastinal invasion, cure by irradiation was unlikely and it would therefore be of more service to the patient to await the development of symptoms the amelioration of which by irradiation would be of more measurable benefit to the patient. On these grounds 35 patients were not managed by irradiation when first they were seen, and a further 13 were not irradiated because they were on general grounds too ill. The remaining patients were irradiated at the time of first assessment, and 16 were later irradiated. Of the 132 patients, 40 had died within six months of first investigation, 61 more within 12 months, and 19 others died during the second year after irradiation. Two patients are at present alive —two and two and a half years after irradiation respectively; 10 patients survived irradiation by longer than two years; these 10 patients have all died, from metastases, the last having survived for five years after irradiation.

From this group of 132 patients it may be said that, when the only clinical evidence of mediastinal invasion is interruption of the left recurrent laryngeal nerve, the primary site of bronchial carcinoma is more likely to be the left lung; that there is a substantial group of patients in whom the diagnosis of bronchial carcinoma must be presumptive—on the grounds of a left pulmonary opacity, often hilar or in the upper lobe, and paralysis of the left vocal cord— without histological confirmation of the diagnosis at the time of first assessment; and that where histological proof of the diagnosis is achieved the tumour is often squamous and may be slow-growing, since survival from the onset of hoarseness of voice may be surprisingly long.

Cord paralysis was demonstrated in a further 100 patients in the series of 4,000—in two patients with Pancoast's syndrome, in four with pulmono-pulmonary metastases, in 11 with superior vena caval obstruction, in 39 with cervical glandular metastases, and in 45 with evidence of tumour spread in several sites. The right vocal cord was paralysed in 19 of this group of 100, and in most of these 19 patients there was a mass of glands in the right side of the neck or a large right supra-hilar, paramediastinal shadow which extended to the root of the neck.

XII. OTHER METASTASES

Cutaneous or subcutaneous metastases were the only evidence of dissemination of bronchial carcinoma in 38 patients and in 19 other patients were found in conjunction with additional clinical evidence of spread. Cutaneous metastases were always small and the patient, in some instances, was sure that the nodule had been present "for years"; in other instances a nodule had been seen to appear and to grow rapidly, and when it had achieved the size of a split pea, to cease to grow. Subcutaneous metastases were generally of the size of a cherry when they were clinically recognised. Cutaneous and subcutaneous metastases were more often felt than seen, and the habit of examining the patient's integument by rubbing the palms of the hands over all the skin surface is recommended.

Metastases in muscle were encountered in only eight patients, and six of these presented because of the appearance of a mass in a muscle—triceps in one, quadriceps in three, calf and rectus abdominis one each. These six patients denied respiratory symptoms even after a primary pulmonary tumour had been demonstrated by routine radiography in the search for a primary. In two patients, both with muscle metastases in the anterior abdominal wall, presentation was with respiratory symptoms.

Metastases in scars were found in three patients and in all were the reason for presentation. The scar of inguinal hernia repair undertaken 30 years earlier; the scar of empyema drainage 20 years earlier; and the scar of laparotomy presumably for appendicectomy 15 years earlier were the sites of metastases which in these three patients constituted the only evidence of dissemination of the pulmonary carcinoma, which was recognised after biopsy of a metastasis and chest radiography, in that order.

Two men presented with purpura, and were found to have splenomegaly; in the course of investigation a pulmonary opacity was seen on chest radiography and sheets of tumour cells were demonstrated in sternal marrow.

An abdominal mass other than hepatic was found in nine patients with established bronchial carcinoma—squamous in four, and undifferentiated in five (" oat-cell " in three of these). In two of these patients the abdominal mass was renal, one of the two had haematuria, and in both the pyelogram was abnormal. The histological features in one of these two cases were those of oat-cell carcinoma and in the other of squamous carcinoma; in both the histologist's opinion was that the bronchial biopsy was from the primary tumour and not from a metastasis from the kidney. Isolated pulmonary metastases from renal carcinoma were encountered as a clinical entity three times during the same period. In one of these last-mentioned three patients the pulmonary lesion, found in the course of investigation of haemoptysis, was associated with an abnormality at bronchoscopy and the bronchoscopic biopsy was confidently reported to show the features of renal carcinoma. The report was unjustifiably disbelieved, and pneumonectomy was undertaken. The resected specimen was again reported to contain a large metastasis from a renal carcinoma; pyelography showed the kidney on the same side as the pneumonectomy to contain a tumour and the kidney was then resected. In the other two instances a peripheral pulmonary lesion was managed as if it had been a peripheral pulmonary carcinoma; examination of the resected specimen

113

showed that the lesion was a metastasis from renal carcinoma and subsequent investigation confirmed that there was a silent renal primary. Chest wall, pleural and multiple pulmonary metastases from renal carcinoma were more common and renal carcinoma is one of the tumours which must be kept constantly in mind during the management of tumours of the chest wall, since these are commonly metastatic, and, especially if they pulsate, commonly metastatic from the kidney.

An abdominal mass in five patients with bronchial carcinoma was established sooner or later to be a suprarenal metastasis. Suprarenal metastases from pulmonary carcinoma are common—but are rarely clinically palpable. A pelvic mass in one woman was established after limited laparotomy and biopsy to be an ovarian metastasis from bronchial carcinoma. A mobile abdominal mass in a man was found after limited laparotomy and biopsy to be a large metastasis in the greater omentum.

Unusual sites of metastases were the scalp (in three patients), the tongue, a tonsil, the hard palate, the lower alveolus, a thumb and a second toe. In none of these nine patients were these unusual metastases the only evidence of tumour spread. The digital metastases presented in such a way as to make a casualty officer believe that he was dealing with chronic paronychia, and the diagnosis was made only when tumour fungated through a surgical incision some weeks later. The scalp metastases were multiple and limited to the scalp in two patients; in one there was a single scalp metastasis managed surgically in the belief that it was a primary integumental tumour, possibly a sebaceous adenoma.

XIII. EVIDENCE AT BRONCHOSCOPY OF UNSUITABILITY FOR SURGICAL MANAGEMENT

In the series of patients with bronchial carcinoma under discussion a tumour was judged unsuitable for surgical management when it was shown that the main carina was invaded or the main carina, while not ulcerated, was unequivocally broad with the main bronchi splayed; when the trachea was involved, unless this involvement was limited to the lateral wall of the trachea on the right, in relation to a tumour in the right upper bronchus; when the trachea was compressed or scabbard-shaped; when tumour could be demonstrated histologically to involve bronchi, usually the main bronchi, of both sides; when tumour obstructed a main bronchus, on the right within $\frac{1}{2}$ cm. of the main carina, and on the left within $1\frac{1}{2}$ cm. of the main carina, provided that involvement at this point was not limited to the lateral wall; and when, by the independent assessment of two experts, a main bronchus was found to be abnormally rigid—an assessment rarely accepted as the only basis for rejecting for surgical management a patient suitable in all other respects. Paralysis of a vocal cord was usually recognised at bronchoscopy but this particular contra-indication has already been considered.

Of 4,000 patients with bronchial carcinoma 179 were not managed surgically because of an endoscopic contra-indication. Of the 179, 25 were women, eight of them in the sixth decade, 11 in the seventh and six in the eighth decade. Two of the women claimed never to have smoked and in two the tumour was an adenocarcinoma—of which there were only two other examples in the group of 179. The three youngest of the 154 men were 27, 28 and 29 years respectively; six men were in the fourth decade, 27 in the fifth, 48 in the sixth, 54 in the seventh, and 16 in the eighth decade. Apart from the four patients with adenocarcinoma, the tumour in 104 was squamous and in 71 undifferentiated (called " oat-cell " in 22 of these)—a proportion of squamous tumours not significantly different from that in this series as a whole.

Four patients with bronchoscopic evidence of unsuitability for surgical management presented with an abnormal routine radiograph made for an unrelated purpose—all had squamous tumours, and one is alive seven years after irradiation. Two patients presented with hypertrophic pulmonary osteoarthropathy. One long survivor has been mentioned; another—a male who smoked heavily and in whom the tumour was an undifferentiated carcinoma— is alive 13 years after irradiation; eight patients died during the third year and seven patients during the second year after irradiation and all the others had died within a year of irradiation, omitting five whose period of survival is not known. Distant metastases were clinically obvious in 53 patients at some time during the interval between completion of irradiation and death; 47 patients are known to have died from asphyxia.

Three patients, who presented with haemoptysis, and in whom at bronchoscopy a tumour was found by its position to be unsuitable for surgical management, had chest radiographs which, even in retrospect, were normal. These three have previously been mentioned. Of the remaining 176 patients in this group the primary tumour was right-sided in 132—a disproportionate emphasis on the right in comparison with the series as a whole. In 12 patients a radiographic lesion on the right was associated with either a scabbard trachea or one so occluded by tumour that more distal vision was precluded even after considerable quantities of tumour had been enucleated at endoscopy to establish an airway. In 14 patients the endoscopically visible lesion was confined to the right main bronchus; in 54 patients a radiographic abnormality, most often in the right upper lobe, but in some in either the right lower lobe or the middle and lower lobes together, was associated with tumour which extended proximally in the right stem bronchus to the main carina, which was ulcerated —and in some of these patients there was an interval of normal-looking bronchial mucosa between the tumour in the lower or intermediate bronchus and that at the main carina; in 18 patients tumour in the right stem bronchus extended to involve the trachea; in 24 patients a right-sided radiographic abnormality was associated with tumour in both main bronchi, at the main carina, and in some also in the posterior tracheal wall; in 10 patients a right-sided radiographic abnormality was associated with an expected bronchoscopic abnormality, such as tumour at the orifice of a bronchus the subtended lobe of which was shrunken, and, in addition tumour in the left stem bronchus, usually on the medial wall and usually in close relation to the main carina, but in two at least 4 cm. distal to the main carina.

In 44 patients the radiographic abnormality was left-sided; in 21 of these tumour occluded the left main bronchus too close to the main carina to allow of successful surgical management; in 10 tumour extended from the left main bronchus to the main carina and in seven others further, to the trachea; and in six the left lower bronchus was occluded by tumour and there was an interval of normal-looking bronchial mucosa between this and tumour at the main carina.

Evidence at bronchoscopy of tumour extension which precluded surgical management on this ground alone was associated, in 12 patients with obstruction of the superior vena cava; in 28 patients with cervical glandular metastases, bilateral in nine of these and ipsilateral in the others; with displacement of the barium-filled oesophagus in 59 patients; and with oesophageal displacement together with other evidence of mediastinal invasion such as phrenic paresis or vocal cord paralysis in 39 patients. In many of the patients in whom tumour extended proximally to the trachea or main carina, or involved both stem bronchi, it was assumed that what was seen at bronchoscopy represented invasion of trachea, main carina and bronchi from mediastinal glands themselves the site of lymph-borne metastases, and it is a little surprising that there were so many patients in whom the only evidence of tumour dissemination was bronchoscopic, and that there were not more with this evidence of dissemination who, in addition, had oesophageal displacement at least, if not phrenic and recurrent laryngeal nerve palsies.

X

Management other than Surgical for Reasons other than Metastases

SUMMARY

Respiratory function in nearly 3 per cent of patients was so poor that surgical management of bronchial carcinoma was precluded on this ground alone. Nearly all were men; 75 per cent were 60 years or older; and, where the cell-type of the tumour was known, most were squamous.

Extensive, active pulmonary tuberculosis, contralateral or bilateral; severe chronic asthma; gross radiographic changes of simple or complicated pneumoconiosis; bullous emphysema and bronchiectasis together precluded surgical management in 35 patients. In 38 patients age alone was regarded as a bar to pulmonary resection—most were men over 75 years. In 27 patients myocardial disease was the only contra-indication to surgical management; 36 patients were so frail that most were unsuitable for any form of treatment. There were occasional other contra-indications to surgical management in patients in whom the pulmonary tumour was judged to be confined to the lung; 2 per cent of patients declined investigation or treatment and a further 2 per cent died before investigations were completed. Two patients died from complications of investigative procedures.

I. PATIENTS IN WHOM THORACOTOMY WAS PRECLUDED BECAUSE OF LIMITATION OF RESPIRATORY FUNCTION

RESPIRATORY function in 115 (2·9 per cent) of 4,000 patients with pulmonary carcinoma was so poor that thoracotomy was precluded. In this group poor function was the only contra-indication to surgical management. Respiratory function in some other patients was shown, because of an enthusiastic determination to complete case records, to be at a level which precluded thoracotomy, but in these patients there was already histological and fluoroscopic proof of tumour spread of an extent which in itself was a bar to operative management.

Of the 115 patients, 112 were men. The three women were all older than 60 years—one was 62, one 67, and the last, who denied ever having smoked, 74 years. The youngest man was 49, 24 were in the sixth decade, 61 in the seventh, and 26 were older than 70 years, the eldest being 78. Of the 112 men, therefore, 23 per cent were older than 69 years, in comparison with 10 per cent in the whole series, and 14 per cent in the latter half of the series. Of the whole series of 3,597 men 48 per cent were older than 59 years, whereas amongst those men in whom function precluded thoracotomy more than 75 per cent were older than 59 years. Amongst the 1,808 men in the second half of the series there was

117

a shift towards an older age group, previously mentioned, but even here only 57 per cent were older than 59 years. In this series, it may therefore be said that impairment of respiratory reserve of a degree which precluded surgical management was commonly related to advanced age—which is precisely what could reasonably be anticipated.

Amongst the group of 115 patients with poor respiratory reserve, histological confirmation of the diagnosis of carcinoma was obtained in 92—by biopsy at bronchoscopy in 68; for the first time at necropsy in 12; by the recognition of malignant cells in sputa in eight others; and by biopsy of cervical glands in four in whom these glands were not enlarged at the time when thoracotomy was excluded as a form of management on the ground of limited respiratory reserve, but in whom cervical nodes became palpable six to eight months later. In 47 patients tumours were peripheral, as opposed to bronchoscopically visible in 68. Histological diagnosis was achieved sooner or later in 24 of these 47 patients with peripheral tumours. It would have been particularly valuable to have obtained the diagnosis of carcinoma from the recognition of cells in sputum in the other 23 patients with peripheral tumours, but repeated examinations were negative. Of the total, the tumour was squamous in 61, undifferentiated in 23, and of unspecified cell type, the cells being recognised in sputa, in eight. In none was the diagnosis of adenocarcinoma made. Histological confirmation of the diagnosis was not achieved in 23 patients, but in two of these a peripheral pulmonary opacity was associated with invasion of the chest wall with radiographic evidence of rib erosion—both patients declined to submit even to aspiration biopsy; and slow but unequivocal growth of the tumour was observed on serial radiographs over six to eight months in seven, in two of whom the lesion was seen radiographically to cavitate. Of the 47 peripheral tumours 13 were cavitated and 18 were smaller than 4 cm. in diameter. Since so many patients with peripheral tumours died before the tumour had reached a large size, and without clinical evidence of metastasis, it is suggested that these patients died with rather than from bronchial carcinoma. Only 20 of 115 patients in this group were seen before 1957. There are several possible reasons for this: the standard of note-taking and records may have improved, but of this there is no other evidence; detailed respiratory function figures were routinely assessed from about 1957 onwards, whereas before this time the assessment of respiratory function was clinical, on the ground of exercise tolerance—a perfectly valid assessment but one which cannot be expressed scientifically as a convenient figure in the same way as can, for example, the forced expiratory volume in a given time; and since limitation of function as a contra-indication to surgical management is commoner in the older age groups, and it has been shown that bronchial carcinoma in this series involved an older age group in the second half of the series, it may be reasoned that more patients in the second half of the series, should be precluded from management by resection.

Seventeen patients were not treated in any way because respiratory reserve was so limited that it was judged that the fibrosis initiated by radiotherapy would make life intolerable; three patients died during the period of investigation, all from coronary insufficiency; the rest were managed by radiotherapy. All but one smoked; three were pipe smokers; one claimed to smoke 100 cigarettes a day. Twenty-seven patients in this group were coal-miners, all with radiographic evidence of pneumoconiosis, 11 with radiographic changes suggestive of progressive massive fibrosis, and most in receipt of pensions ranging from 20 to 50 per cent from the Coal Board.

Two patients in this group are alive five years after irradiation. In one a tumour was seen to occlude the lower part of the right main bronchus and was shown by biopsy to be squamous in type; the middle and lower lobes were shrunken and airless; following irradiation the shrunken lobes slowly became aerated, and have remained so, although occupying a smaller than normal volume of the hemithorax; the present bronchoscopic appearances are those of stricture of the bronchus at the level of the earlier biopsy, but with a lumen reduced only by about half its expected diameter, and without gross or microscopic evidence of tumour recurrence; respiratory function has deteriorated a little further. The second five year survivor, one of seven patients who presented following the detection at routine mass miniature radiography of a pulmonary shadow, is discussed in Chapter VII.

One patient died two years and two months after radiotherapy; death was sudden during an acute illness and was shown at necropsy to be the consequence of acute haemorrhagic pancreatitis; there were small hepatic metastases from bronchial carcinoma, of which there was no residual evidence in the lung, although irradiation fibrosis was described as extensive. All the other patients in this group have died, most within six months of first attendance at hospital, all but four within a year, and all within 18 months.

II. OTHER NON-METASTATIC CONTRA-INDICATIONS

1. Pulmonary Tuberculosis. Bronchial carcinoma in 14 patients, all of them men, was not managed surgically because in each it was associated with extensive active pulmonary tuberculosis—bilateral in three and contralateral and cavitated in 11. The tumour in nine of the 14 patients in this group was squamous and in five undifferentiated (" oat-cell " in two of these). All but one were in the sixth or seventh decade—the exception was a youth of 19 years who died within five months of the diagnosis of carcinoma of the bronchus and pulmonary tuberculosis having been made, and who, at post-mortem examination was established to have had an undifferentiated tumour which widely invaded the mediastinum together with extensive bilateral cavitated tuberculosis. Two patients died two and two and a half years after the diagnosis had been established, and the rest died within a year.

2. Asthma. Six men, all in the sixth or seventh decade and all with bronchoscopically visible squamous tumours, were not treated in any way because of severe asthma. Two of these men denied ever having smoked. One died three years after the diagnosis of carcinoma had been established; the others died within 18 months.

119

3. Pneumoconiosis. Radiographic changes of pneumoconiosis or progressive massive fibrosis were regarded as of such an extent to constitute a bar to surgical or radiotherapeutic management of bronchial carcinoma in eight patients, all with bronchoscopically visible squamous tumours, despite failure to demonstrate, by measurement of respiratory function, limitation of respiratory reserve of a degree which alone constituted a contra-indication to surgical management. Two of these patients survived for two and a half years; the others died within a year of investigation.

4. Bullous Emphysema. In four men the radiographic appearances of bullous emphysema, bilateral in three and contralateral in one, were regarded as of an extent which precluded surgical or radiotherapeutic management of bronchial carcinoma despite respiratory reserve which, by measurement, was not in itself prohibitively low. In one of these four patients the diagnosis of carcinoma was presumptive until, seven months later, a cervical node became palpable; the three in whom the tumour was visible at bronchoscopy all had squamous tumours and none survived longer than a year.

5. Bronchiectasis. A man of 54 years who denied ever having smoked and who had been shown 10 years earlier to have extensive bilateral bronchiectasis outwith safe limits of surgical management was shown, after investigation of haemoptysis, which was a new symptom to him, to have a squamous tumour in the right upper bronchus. A man of 71 years who had previously been submitted to middle and lower lobectomy for bronchiectasis was found to have an " oat-cell " carcinoma of the contralateral lower bronchus eight years later. A woman of 49 years, investigated for haemoptysis, was shown to have an undifferentiated carcinoma of the bronchus and a bronchogram was made to try to explain contralateral radiographic honeycombing; extensive bilateral bronchiectasis was demonstrated. Management in these three patients was by irradiation and none survived longer than 18 months.

Carcinoma and bronchiectasis co-existed in the resected lung in three of 78 patients in whom total unilateral bronchiectasis was managed by pneumonectomy. In two men of 41 and 43 years respectively, in neither of whom the diagnosis of carcinoma was suspected pre-operatively, the tumour was squamous and both are alive, 10 and 12 years after pneumonectomy, one with cor pulmonale. The third carcinoma was undifferentiated and was found in a lung resected from a 19-year-old girl who did not smoke and who is well 13 years later. Abnormal clumps of epithelial cells which produced tumour-like formations and which are called tumourlets are found in 20 per cent of lobes or lungs resected for bronchiectasis; the carcinomata in these cases were histologically distinct from tumourlets.

Two men, earlier shown to have right upper bronchiectasis, and regarded as patients who did not require surgical management because of their age and relative paucity of symptoms, later developed right upper squamous tumours of central type—one three and one nine years after initial investigation. Both were managed by pneumonectomy and both are alive; in neither was there glandular metastasis.

120

6. Age. In 38 patients age was accepted as the only contra-indication to surgical management of bronchial carcinoma. Of the 38 patients 35 were men. Chronological age alone is difficult to define as a bar to surgical management— if 80 is too old, is 79 also too old? The relationship between age and post-operative mortality amongst patients in whom bronchial carcinoma was managed by resection has already been presented in detail and there is no doubt that a higher proportion of older patients die in convalescence from pulmonary resection. Of the 38 patients regarded as too old for surgical management, 30 were 75 years or older and four were 80 years old. Most were not only chronologically but also physiologically old—two patients of 80 years were, however, in remarkably good physiological condition. The diagnosis of carcinoma was histologically established in 32—in 22 the tumour was squamous and in 10 undifferentiated; in six the tumour was peripheral and the diagnosis was presumptive. All these patients had died five months to two and a half years from the time of investigation, and it is the impression that some at least died with rather than from bronchial carcinoma. Of the 38, 17 were managed by radiotherapy.

7. Myocardial disease. In 27 patients myocardial disease was accepted as the only contra-indication to surgical management of bronchial carcinoma— congestive cardiac failure in six; recent myocardial infarction in nine (with a history of previous infarction in four of these), and angina in 12. In seven other patients an abnormality of cardiac rhythm developed in close relation to investigation of bronchial carcinoma. All were submitted to thoracotomy. In four atrial invasion was of such an extent that resection was technically impossible; in two there was atrial invasion but pneumonectomy with control of the pulmonary veins at atrial level was undertaken; in one there was an isolated metastasis in the ventricular wall as well as atrial invasion; and in the last there was no evidence of cardiac invasion. It may be that the development of a cardiac arrhythmia constitutes a valid contra-indication to surgical management of bronchial carcinoma.

Of the 27 patients with myocardial disease histological confirmation of the diagnosis of bronchial carcinoma was achieved in all of them—in five only at necropsy. In 13 the tumour was a squamous carcinoma and in 13 an undifferentiated carcinoma (" oat-cell " in two of these); in one, in whom histological confirmation of the diagnosis of carcinoma was achieved only at necropsy, the tumour was an adenocarcinoma. Three of the 27 patients were women; the youngest in the group was a man of 50 years and only four were younger than 65 years.

8. Frailty. In the case records of 36 patients, all with histologically established bronchial carcinoma and without clinical, radiographic, fluoroscopic or bronchoscopic evidence of dissemination of tumour, the statement was made that although measurement of respiratory function did not preclude management of bronchial carcinoma by resection, " frailty " (or in some instances " decrepitude ") was such that, on general grounds, these patients were all regarded as unsuitable for surgical management—and indeed in some instances for treatment of any sort. The youngest patient in this group of 36 was 55; most were older than 65 years and the three oldest were 71; three were women. In 24 the tumour was squamous and in 12 undifferentiated. These patients were all discharged from hospital and died at home within six months of investigation. In none did the opportunity again arise for examination in the Thoracic Unit, and in none was a post-mortem examination undertaken, so that it is not possible to relate frailty in these patients to cryptic metastasis or other disease of a degenerative nature.

9. Unusual Non-Metastatic Contra-Indications. A man of 78 who, in the eight preceding years had been submitted to both oesophagectomy for squamous carcinoma and resection of an abdominal aortic aneurysm with restoration of aortic continuity with a dacron prosthesis, presented with a squamous carcinoma in the right upper bronchus. The tumour was small; there was no reason to call it anything other than bronchial carcinoma and there was no evidence of extra-pulmonary spread. It seemed unfair again to submit him to another major operation and management was by irradiation. He died eight months later from coronary thrombosis without evidence of tumour anywhere at necropsy.

A man of 43 with haemophilia was seen at bronchoscopy—undertaken because of chest pain and shrinkage of the middle lobe—to have a nodular lesion which obstructed the middle bronchus; a biopsy was not made for fear of precipitating severe haemorrhage and management was by irradiation. He is well 10 years later and the radiographic changes are only those of irradiation fibrosis. In him the diagnosis of bronchial carcinoma is based only on macroscopic evidence.

A man of 55 developed haemoptysis while encased in a plaster jacket because of traumatic fracture of a dorsal vertebra. The trauma was gross; there was no reason to believe that the fracture was pathological and its subsequent behaviour confirmed that the vertebral lesion was only traumatic. He was shown to have an undifferentiated carcinoma of the left lower bronchus and was managed by irradiation because of the difficulty of management by thoracotomy in the circumstances.

A man of 56 with a squamous carcinoma bronchoscopically visible is recorded as having been irradiated because he had, in addition, syringomyelia.

A man of 56 with an " oat-cell " carcinoma without clinical or other evidence of spread was accepted by surgeons and radiotherapists alike as suitable for management, and management by irradiation was offered after reference to the Medical Research Council who were conducting a trial on the results of management of " oat-cell " carcinoma.[1]

III. PATIENTS WHO DECLINED INVESTIGATION OR TREATMENT

Of 4,000 patients with bronchial carcinoma 80 (2 per cent) declined investigation or treatment. Of the 80 only three were women. Of the 77 men

[1] Medical Research Council Working-party (1966). *Lancet*, 2, 979.

56 were in the seventh or eighth decade and the two youngest were 45 and 48 years respectively. In 35 patients the tumour was a squamous carcinoma (five of these patients presented with an abnormal mass radiograph and denied respiratory symptoms), in six the tumour was an undifferentiated carcinoma (" oat-cell " in one), in 27 the appearances at bronchoscopy were normal and histological confirmation of the diagnosis was not obtained, and 12 patients declined to submit even to bronchoscopy so that the opportunity for making a histological diagnosis was denied.

On the basis of clinical examination and chest radiography in all 80 patients, and on the additional evidence of fluoroscopy and bronchoscopy in 68 of the 80 patients, the tumours in this group were surgically manageable. Four of the men were older than 75 years, and if they had stayed long enough in hospital for formal discussion of management, they would probably have been referred for management by irradiation rather than by exploratory thoracotomy. One of these men, with an undifferentiated tumour, denied ever having smoked—he died six months later. The others were regarded as suitable candidates for management by exploration with a view to pulmonary resection, and all in whom investigation had been completed were offered this form of management. All declined surgical management, and 17, who either accepted irradiation as an alternative form of management when offered this, or asked to be managed in this way before being offered the alternative, were irradiated. The remainder either declined management of any sort, or—in three instances —were regarded as unsuitable for irradiation because the bulk of the tumour was such that the whole lesion could not be irradiated and symptoms were minimal. Three of those irradiated are alive, three, four and six years after treatment; four died three or four years after irradiation, one after irradiation for a second time; the remainder died 11 to 27 months after irradiation.

Of the 63 patients who were not treated in any way 19 had died within six months and a further 17 within a year of investigation. Two patients died 15 months and one two years after irradiation; 23 patients in this group cannot be traced—all of them seen before 1954 and 16 of the 23 younger than 60 years at the time that they were investigated. Failure to trace these patients is probably related to a change of general practitioner; it is not known what significance to attach to the relative youth of this group except to relate it to the observation made earlier that bronchial carcinoma in the first half of the series affected a higher percentage of younger people.

IV. DEATH BEFORE COMPLETION OF INVESTIGATIONS

Investigations were incomplete in 74 patients at the time of death. Of these 74 patients nine were women. The two youngest women—of 34 and 37 years respectively—were admitted for the investigation of a pulmonary opacity found during the investigation of a profound and rapidly advancing neuropathy; both died from fulminating pulmonary infection probably unrelated to the pulmonary carcinoma—in both an undifferentiated tumour—which was demonstrated at necropsy. Carcinomatous neuropathy or myopathy was

123

recognised in only five other patients in the series. All seven patients presented with symptoms not of pulmonary disease but of the muscular or neural conco-mitants, and all died within two months of the diagnosis of pulmonary carcinoma having been established or suggested, none being regarded as a suitable candidate for any form of treatment. One of these patients had hyper-trophic pulmonary osteo-arthropathy.

Of the 74 patients who died before investigation was complete 29 died suddenly, five from pulmonary embolism—a diagnosis substantiated in all at necropsy—and 24 as if from myocardial infarction—a diagnosis established in only seven at necropsy. Although there had not been found clinical evidence of dissemination of tumour in these 29 patients, there was in all of them at necropsy evidence of tumour spread of an extent which would have made treatment of any sort pointless. In eight of those who died suddenly and in whom the diagnosis of myocardial infarction was suggested, extensive cardiac invasion by the pulmonary tumour was demonstrated.

Eleven patients were found, at the time of admission, to have good evidence of bronchial carcinoma but also to be in severe congestive cardiac failure from which they died sooner or later, never having been made well enough for further investigation of the pulmonary lesion. In all the diagnosis of bronchial carcinoma was confirmed at necropsy. Death from cor pulmonale in five other patients during the course of investigation is recorded in the notes, and the diagnosis of carcinoma is, in these, confirmed histologically but there is no necropsy record. An acute cerebral episode in six patients was regarded clinically as evidence of cerebral metastasis but at necropsy was shown to be the conse-quence of a cerebral vascular accident.

Sixteen patients were admitted so ill that they were never suitable even for bronchoscopy and, although in none of them was there evidence of dissemi-nation of tumour on clinical examination, all had widespread tumour at necropsy, and all had suprarenal metastases. Three patients died from massive haemoptysis shortly after admission and before investigation was undertaken. In these carcinomatous invasion of a large pulmonary vessel was demonstrated at necropsy.

Two patients died from investigative procedures—one from haemorrhage the consequence of a biopsy made at bronchoscopy, and in him it was confirmed that the biopsy had been from a carina; the other died during thoracentesis for pleural effusion associated with bronchial carcinoma, and it was thought that death may have been from air embolism, but this was never confirmed.

XI

Management in Special Circumstances

SUMMARY

In 3·3 per cent of patients bronchial carcinoma was found to invade the chest wall. In a third of these a resection was undertaken because chest wall invasion was lateral; in another third the tumour was apical and associated with the features of Pancoast's syndrome; in the last third invasion was medial, either anterior or posterior. An attempt was not made surgically to manage apical tumours with Pancoast's syndrome or tumours which invaded medially.

Pleural effusion as an accompaniment of bronchial carcinoma was routinely investigated by thoracoscopy, a technique which demonstrated the presence of pleural metastases as the only evidence of extra-pulmonary extension of bronchial carcinoma in 2·1 per cent of patients. Half the number of patients with pleural metastases had peripheral tumours, and a quarter were women. Adenocarcinoma disseminated to the pleural space disproportionately often. Most patients with pleural metastases had died within six months of the diagnosis having been made. Pleural effusion, even if sanguinous, in association with bronchial carcinoma is not synonymous with pleural metastasis and is no more than an indication for further investigation.

Empyema thoracis was related to bronchial carcinoma or complicated an operation for bronchial carcinoma in 1·4 per cent of patients. Thoracoplasty is not usually required in the management of post-pneumonectomy empyema. Where empyema complicated pulmonary resection for bronchial carcinoma, survival time was sometimes surprisingly long.

Hypertrophic pulmonary osteo-arthropathy was present in 1·2 per cent of patients with bronchial carcinoma; in more than two-thirds the tumour was resected and in more than two-thirds the tumour was peripheral. A disproportionately large number of tumours were adenocarcinomata, and, despite the high operability rate, long survival was achieved only half as often as in patients who did not have hypertrophic pulmonary osteo-arthropathy. Resection of the primary tumour relieved joint pain in all patients.

I. BRONCHIAL CARCINOMA WITH INVASION OF THE CHEST WALL

OF 4,000 patients with bronchial carcinoma the primary pulmonary tumour at the time of first investigation invaded directly the adjacent chest wall in 131. In 45 of these patients invasion was lateral to the posterior rib angle, did not involve the first rib or sternum, and was associated at exploratory thoracotomy with a pulmonary tumour amenable to resection; in these 45 patients resection was completed—by pneumonectomy in 27 and lobectomy in 18—with resection of part of the chest wall (le Roux, 1964.)[1] In

[1] Le Roux, B. T. (1964). Maintenance of chest wall stability. *Thorax*, **19**, 397.

125

37 patients with bronchial carcinoma with chest wall invasion the tumour was apical and invaded also the brachial plexus and the cervical sympathetic —these patients are discussed in the section devoted to Pancoast's syndrome. In 49 patients bronchial carcinoma was associated with chest wall invasion of an extent or at a site where resection was regarded as so unlikely to be technically possible that management was other than surgical.

Of the last mentioned 49 patients invasion of the chest wall in 25 was demonstrated radiographically to involve one or more ribs medial to the posterior rib angle. In eight patients invasion of similar extent and situation was associated with a palpable mass in a scapulo-vertebral interval and in six patients there was a mass inseparable from the chest wall palpable in the axilla; seven of the last mentioned 14 patients presented with the complaints of pain and a chest wall swelling. In 10 patients the chest wall invasion was anterior and involved the sternum and adjacent costal cartilages. The tumours in all these patients were peripheral in type and histological confirmation of the diagnosis of carcinoma—squamous in 27 and undifferentiated in 14—was achieved in 41 by either aspiration biopsy or biopsy through a limited incision. In eight patients the radiographic appearances were accepted as sufficiently strong evidence of the diagnosis of bronchial carcinoma for management by irradiation to be undertaken without histological confirmation.

In the group of 131 patients with chest wall invasion of pulmonary carcinoma only two were women. The youngest was a man of 43 who claimed never to have smoked; in him the tumour was an undifferentiated carcinoma and he died two months after investigation.

Seven patients who presented with respiratory symptoms and a peripheral pulmonary shadow regarded as most likely to be a pulmonary carcinoma and declined surgical management returned within a year of first investigation with chest pain and the radiographic features of chest wall invasion. One of the seven patients was managed surgically and five others were irradiated. The last still declined treatment of any sort; in him pain disappeared spontaneously and he survived a further 18 months and died apparently from coronary thrombosis.

Pancoast's Syndrome. Of 4,000 patients with pulmonary carcinoma, the tumour in 37 (0·9 per cent) was peripheral in type, situated at the right pulmonary apex in 23 and at the left in 14, and associated with ipsilateral Horner's syndrome, wasting of the small muscles of the hand, pain in the arm and erosion of some or all of the highest three ribs. In one patient there was, in addition, vertebral erosion; in two patients the ipsilateral pupil was dilated at the time of admission but contracted within a few days. All presented because of the symptoms associated with parietal invasion; the additional clinical features of superior vena caval obstruction were present in two at the time of admission, and two patients, one with superior vena caval obstruction, were hoarse of voice; two patients had had haemoptysis and four recognised the recent onset of dyspnoea. All complained of pain varying in duration from two to 18 months.

Of the 37 patients with Pancoast's syndrome only two were women, neither of whom smoked; both were younger than 40 years, and one was five months pregnant—in her, histological confirmation of the diagnosis was achieved by cervical gland biopsy, and the tumour was squamous in type. Of the 35 men, two were younger than 40 years, two others younger than 50, 15 were in the sixth decade and 12 in the seventh decade, and four were older than 70, the oldest being 75 years. The youngest patient in the whole group was a woman of 32 years.

Histological confirmation of the diagnosis was achieved in 20 patients. In 16 cervical glandular metastases, in all ipsilateral, were clinically palpable and confirmed histologically; in four others histological confirmation was achieved, by aspiration biopsy in two, and by limited posterior thoracotomy with biopsy of an invaded rib in two. Of these 20 patients the tumour was squamous in 14 and undifferentiated in six (one " oat-celled "). In five other patients the neck was explored and the scalene node removed was not shown to contain tumour. In all, the bronchoscopic appearances were normal.

In three patients the ipsilateral phrenic nerve was paralysed and in two the barium-filled oesophagus was seen to be displaced. The cord palsy was left-sided in one of the two patients who were hoarse, and right-sided in the other, this patient having in addition to a right Pancoast's syndrome, hoarseness of voice and superior vena caval obstruction, right phrenic paresis, oesophageal displacement and cervical lymph-glandular metastases.

Management in all but one patient, who was considered too ill for any form of treatment, was by irradiation. Of the 37 patients 34 have died, all within a year of admission to hospital and 16 within six months of admission. Three are alive —the 32-year-old female, two years after irradiation, a 71-year-old man two and a half years after irradiation, and a 56-year-old man five years after irradiation. In none of the three who are at present alive was histological confirmation of the diagnosis achieved. Two patients required leucotomy for pain unrelieved by radiotherapy; in the others relief of pain was achieved but pain returned in several in the weeks which preceded death; superior vena caval obstruction was relieved by irradiation in the two patients with this syndrome. In one of these and in three other patients superior vena caval obstruction was present at the time of death.

In the 15-year period under discussion one patient, a man of 34, presented with Horner's syndrome and pain in the arm, an apical radiographic opacity with a well-defined caudal margin, and a boggy swelling in the neck. The syndrome was of recent onset, the small muscles of the hand were not wasted, and the presenting syndrome included fever. He was thought most likely to have a rapidly growing tumour. The neck was explored and pus was found in the retro-pharyngeal space. A year later he was well, still with Horner's syndrome.

II. BRONCHIAL CARCINOMA WITH PLEURAL EFFUSION

In the period under discussion pleural effusion was routinely investigated in this Unit by aspiration of the pleural liquid and its replacement with air; at this juncture postero-anterior and lateral chest radiographs were made; thereafter the pleural surfaces were examined with the thoracoscope and appropriate biopsies were made. It was occasionally possible to demonstrate pleural metastases on plain films after air replacement, thereby providing a visual record of the diagnosis, and it has been demonstrated that biopsy at thoracoscopy is more often informative than that made blindly percutaneously with one of the needles designed for this purpose—simply by making such a biopsy as a preliminary to the insertion of the cannula for thoracoscopy.

Of 4,000 patients with bronchial carcinoma, 82 in whom there was clinical and radiographic evidence of pleural effusion were shown, by the technique outlined above, to have metastases on the parietal pleural surface. This group of patients did not have other evidence of dissemination of tumour. Of the 82 patients 23, or more than a quarter, were women—a proportion so high that the records have been scrutinised with particular care to ensure that in this group of women are not included any whose primary tumour was not pulmonary, and there is no evidence that this error has been made. The youngest of the 23 women was 46 years, 13 were in the sixth decade and the oldest was 83; four women, two with undifferentiated and two with squamous tumours, denied ever having smoked. Of the 59 men, the youngest was 32 years, the oldest 82, and 45 were in the sixth and seventh decades together.

In 42 of the 82 patients the appearances at bronchoscopy were normal or the appearances were those simply of external compression of bronchi, the consequence of the bulk of the effusion—an appearance rarely accepted as final, since it was standard practice to examine the bronchi only after the effusion had been aspirated. In the remaining 40 patients histological confirmation of the diagnosis of bronchial carcinoma was achieved by biopsy of a bronchial abnormality at bronchoscopy. In all patients in whom pleural and bronchial biopsies were positive the histological appearances of these two biopsies were similar.

In 41 patients the tumour was squamous in type; in 34 the tumour was called undifferentiated ("oat-cell" in five of these), and in seven the tumour was an adenocarcinoma. Therefore, not only is the number of women in this group of patients unusually high, but so also is the incidence of adenocarcinoma, relative to its incidence in the series as a whole.

During the first half of the 15-year period under discussion some patients with pleural metastases from bronchial carcinoma were managed by irradiation; latterly this form of treatment has not been adopted since it so rarely proved effective. It is usually possible to depress the rate of re-accumulation of pleural liquid by the instillation of mustine (nitrogen mustard) into the pleural space. Of the 82 patients in this group one died three years after the diagnosis of pleural metastases had been established, and one 18 months later; all the other patients had died within a year of investigation, and most within six months. One patient had presented only because of an abnormality detected at mass radiography.

Pleural effusion in three patients with bronchial carcinoma and superior vena caval obstruction and in 17 patients with cervical glandular metastases from bronchial carcinoma was investigated by thoracoscopy and shown to be related to pleural metastases. Pleural effusion in 43 other patients with clinical, radiographic or fluoroscopic evidence of dissemination of bronchial carcinoma was similarly investigated and pleural metastases were not demonstrated. Pleural effusion is recorded in 62 patients with clinical evidence of dissemination of tumour in whom the effusion was not investigated—and the number of patients with pleural effusion, not investigated because it was of purely academic interest whether or not there were pleural metastases, may well be higher. Pleural effusion in 57 patients in whom this accompaniment of bronchial carcinoma might have constituted a bar to surgical management of the tumour was investigated by thoracoscopy and pleural metastases were not found. These patients were thereupon managed by exploratory thoracotomy. Of the 57, the tumour was irresectable in seven because of mediastinal invasion, five have lived for longer than five years and three are alive less than five years after pulmonary resection, and the rest have died from metastases nine months to seven years after pulmonary resection—an incidence of death from metastases, of survival, and of inoperability in no way different from that in patients who did not have pleural effusion as an accompaniment of bronchial carcinoma when first they were investigated. There is a group of patients—from the records, 43, but it is felt that this figure should be higher—in whom pleural effusion was not recognised on pre-operative radiographs and in whom, at exploratory thoracotomy, pleural liquid in quantity sufficient to arouse comment was found. In this group of 43 patients the tumour was irresectable in only three. Pleural liquid found in these circumstances was collected for histological examination; the recognition of tumour cells in the liquid seems, from the signatures of the reports, to have been limited to two of several examining pathologists; two of seven patients in whose pleural liquid tumour cells were seen have lived longer than five years, and the other five have died from metastases; all but two of the patients in whose pleural liquid tumour cells were not seen have died from metastases.

From the operative records, 23 patients were found at exploratory thoracotomy to have pleural metastases—isolated in seven and diffuse in 16. In the operative record of eight of these 23 patients it is specifically stated that there was no pleural effusion, and reference to pleural effusion in the rest is not made. In none of these patients was a resection made, although in all it was technically possible, since pulmonary resection in the presence of pleural metastases seemed pointless. None survived longer than six months.

The known incidence of pleural metastases at the time of death, as opposed to the time of investigation, in 4,000 patients is 287 (7 per cent), and may well have been higher, since many patients died at home without necropsy. Of all patients with metastatic pleural tumour, 80 per cent died within six months of diagnosis—behaviour significantly different from those with primary pleural

129

tumours. The commonest pleural tumour is a metastasis, and the commonest source of such a metastasis is a primary tumour in the lung (le Roux, 1962).[1]

Experience in this Unit of bronchial carcinoma with related pleural effusion makes it clear that pleural effusion as an accompaniment of bronchial carcinoma, even if the liquid is sanguinous, is not necessarily evidence of pleural invasion by tumour; that the examination of the pleural surfaces through a thoracoscope after replacement of the effusion with air offers the opportunity of making a biopsy of more appropriate tissue than that obtained blindly percutaneously; that survival of patients with bronchial carcinoma with pleural metastases is seldom longer than six months; that the survival rate from pulmonary resection in patients with pleural effusion not associated with pleural metastases does not differ from the survival rate in those without pleural effusion; and finally that pleural effusion as an accompaniment of bronchial carcinoma offers the opportunity for further investigation and is not a reason for despair.

III. BRONCHIAL CARCINOMA WITH EMPYEMA

Of 4,000 patients with pulmonary carcinoma empyema was related to the primary tumour or complicated an operation for carcinoma in 54 (le Roux, 1965).[2] Of 2,217 patients in whom bronchial carcinoma was regarded as unsuitable for surgery—because of evidence of tumour dissemination adduced from routine investigation or because of related lesions which in general made a patient unsuitable for exploratory thoracotomy—empyema co-existed in 18. In eight of these the empyema was managed by closed and in 10 by open drainage. In five patients in whom empyema was managed by open drainage bronchial carcinoma was not suspected as the cause of the empyema and in these the diagnosis of carcinoma was established after histological examination of parietal pleura, a biopsy of which is made routinely at open drainage of empyema thoracis by rib resection. Radiotherapy in these five patients was followed by survival from six to 18 months, but in only one did the empyema heal. In 13 patients empyema complicated extensive bronchial carcinoma, from which these patients died all within 12 weeks of admission to hospital. In eight of these 13 admission was for the investigation of pulmonary disease, probably carcinoma, and empyema was an unexpected finding during the course of routine investigation which established the diagnosis of bronchial carcinoma. In five, admission to hospital was for the management of established empyema, during investigation of the cause of which a bronchial carcinoma was found—at bronchoscopy, or from the histological examination of distant metastatic lesions.

In the 319 patients in whom exploratory thoracotomy was undertaken and the pulmonary tumour was found to be outwith the range of surgical management empyema complicated convalescence in one patient and contributed to death in the post-operative period.

In nine patients bronchial carcinoma and empyema were found, either

[1] Le Roux, B. T. (1962). Pleural tumours. *Thorax*, **17**, 111.
[2] Le Roux, B. T. (1965). Empyema thoracis. *Br. J. Surg.*, **52**, 89.

during routine investigation or at operation, to coexist; in this group of patients evidence of dissemination of tumour outwith the lung was not found, and pulmonary resection, pneumonectomy in seven and lobectomy in two, was undertaken and at the same time the empyema was resected. Empyema recurred post-operatively in one patient who had been submitted to lobectomy and in one submitted to pneumonectomy. In both, post-operative empyema was managed by open drainage, followed, in the patient in whom empyema complicated pneumonectomy, by thoracoplasty. In this group of nine patients the tumour was undifferentiated in two and squamous in seven. Three patients died from metastasis 12, 17 and 19 months respectively after operation; and six, including the two with post-operative empyema, are alive three to nine years after resection. One of these patients, who has now survived operation for nearly seven years, was found at thoracotomy to have histologically substantiated mediastinal lymph-glandular metastases. Six of the tumours were central in type and three peripheral. Those patients still alive all had squamous tumours.

Empyema complicated lobectomy for carcinoma in three patients. Two of the patients who died after lobectomy for carcinoma did so with empyema; the third post-lobectomy empyema was managed by rib resection and the patient is alive five years later; in him the tumour was a peripheral adenocarcinoma.

Empyema complicated pneumonectomy for carcinoma in 23 patients. Of those patients who died directly as a consequence of pneumonectomy, seven did so with empyema, all seven having at some stage during convalescence a bronchopleural fistula. At necropsy in three of these disruption of the bronchial closure was demonstrated, but in the other four a fistula either had healed or was not recognised. Empyema in four of these patients was managed by closed and in three by open drainage.

One patient, in whom empyema complicated pneumonectomy, was managed by open drainage and then discharged from hospital with the drainage tube in situ, the object being to readmit him at a later date for thoracoplasty. He became quickly accustomed to life with a discharging sinus and declined to return to hospital. He lived comfortably for 18 months and when he requested readmission to hospital because he felt less well, he was found to have obstruction of the superior vena cava and cervical lymph-glandular metastases. Despite temporary relief of symptoms by radiotherapy he continued to decline and died from progress of this tumour less than two years after pneumonectomy.

In six patients open drainage of post-pneumonectomy empyema was followed by an extensive thoracoplasty; all these patients were managed before 1955. In nine patients open drainage of post-pneumonectomy empyema was temporary, the drainage tube being retained for only five to 12 days, and the parietal sinus was then allowed to heal. In only one of these patients was revision of drainage required, following which empyema is not known to have recurred. Inadequate closure of the bronchial stump was not demonstrated or suspected in any of these 15 patients.

Two patients in whom post-pneumonectomy empyema was managed by open drainage and thoracoplasty in 1952, and two similarly managed in 1954, are alive: two of these had mediastinal lymph-glandular metastases at operation and in all four the primary tumour was squamous. The two remaining patients managed in this way died from tumour recurrence three and four years after operation: in one the tumour was undifferentiated and in one squamous.

Of the nine patients managed by temporary open drainage six are alive three to seven and a half years after pneumonectomy, and one of these, with an undifferentiated tumour, had mediastinal glandular metastases; three, all with undifferentiated tumours with mediastinal glandular metastases at operation, have died. From these figures it is not possible strongly to support the belief that empyema which complicates pneumonectomy is conducive to longer than average survival, since the number of patients is too small and any increase in their average survival time in comparison with that of patients in whom pneumonectomy was not complicated by empyema, whether or not mediastinal glands were invaded, is not long enough to be significant. It can only be recorded that survival in some of these patients is long and continues, and that, in some, length of survival is a little surprising.

IV. BRONCHIAL CARCINOMA WITH HYPERTROPHIC PULMONARY OSTEOARTHROPATHY

Of 4,000 patients with bronchial carcinoma 49 (1·2 per cent) presented with the clinical features of hypertrophic pulmonary osteoarthropathy. Yacoub (1965)[1] has reviewed the literature on this aspect of pulmonary carcinoma and found the reported incidence of hypertrophic pulmonary osteoarthropathy to vary from 2 per cent to 48 per cent. Joint pain and swelling were the only symptoms to which 32 of the 49 patients admitted; additional symptoms were recognised in 17 patients—dyspnoea of recent onset in eight; haemoptysis in seven; and recurrent febrile illness with pleural pain in two. All but one were men. The woman was 55 years of age; the two youngest men were 37 and 38 years; 10 others were younger than 50; nearly half the total number (23) were between 50 and 59 years; 13 were 60 years or older, the two oldest being 72. All but one smoked; the non-smoker, who claimed never to have smoked, was a man of 58 years with a peripheral squamous tumour which was managed by pneumonectomy; mediastinal glands were not invaded; the clinical features of raised intra-cranial pressure developed two years after pneumonectomy, were attributed to cerebral metastases and were relieved by irradiation; these symptoms recurred late in the third year after pneumonectomy and he died in status epilepticus.

The tumour was visible at bronchoscopy in 15 of the 49 patients and was peripheral in type in the rest, in whom the bronchoscopic appearances were normal. In 25 patients the histological features were those of a squamous

[1] Yacoub, M. W. (1965). Relation between the histology of bronchial carcinoma and hypertrophic pulmonary osteoarthropathy. *Thorax*, **20**, 537.

tumour, in 13 of an undifferentiated tumour, called "oat-cell" in one, and in 11 of an adenocarcinoma—an incidence of adenocarcinoma of 22 per cent; Yacoub (1965)[1] reported an incidence of adenocarcinoma of 30 per cent in patients with hypertrophic pulmonary osteoarthropathy and found none with an "oat-cell" tumour. Resection was undertaken in 34 patients—by pneumonectomy in 24, by lobectomy in nine and by segmental resection in one. In one patient the tumour was found to be irresectable at thoracotomy and in 12 exploratory thoracotomy was not undertaken—in one because the patient, who also had a carcinomatous neuropathy, was judged too ill on general grounds to withstand thoracotomy; in four because of histologically proven cervical glandular metastases (ipsilateral in three and contralateral—from a primary in the left upper lobe to a gland in the right side of the neck—in one in whom the liver was also enlarged and nodular); in two because the tumour was seen at bronchoscopy to lie too close to the tracheal bifurcation; in two because of displacement of the barium-filled oesophagus and in three because of paradoxical movement of a diaphragmatic dome at fluoroscopy. The remaining two patients died, one while awaiting a decision on surgical management, and one, who declined any form of treatment, shortly after returning home, both suddenly, and perhaps from pulmonary embolism, but without necropsy evidence.

The symptoms of hypertrophic pulmonary osteoarthropathy were relieved, in all patients in whom a resection was undertaken, from the moment of recovery from anaesthesia, and by ipsilateral vagotomy in the patient in whom the tumour was found to be irresectable. Irradiation of the pulmonary primary in nine patients relieved pain within a fortnight of the inception of treatment; pain in three patients considered unsuitable for management even by irradiation was imperfectly controlled with increasing doses of morphia.

Radiological evidence of regression of new bone formation and photographic evidence of regression of finger clubbing were recorded in three patients, two managed by pneumonectomy and one by lobectomy. Long bones in relation to the wrists and elbows, ankles and knees were radiographed in nearly all patients before operation and in the three above-mentioned patients before operation and two, four and six months after operation. In all three regression of new bone formation on radiographs made two months after operation was clear, but new bone formation was unmistakable on these films; at four months new bone formation was distinguishable in two but recognisable in the third only by two of four independent expert observers who were denied access to previous films; at six months new bone formation was not recognisable in two patients and appreciable, although greatly diminished, in the ulnae of the third patient.

Only four of the 49 patients with hypertrophic pulmonary osteoarthropathy are alive—one (a pipe-smoker with a squamous tumour without mediastinal glandular metastases) two years after pneumonectomy; one (with

[1] Yacoub, M. W. (1965). Relation between the histology of bronchial carcinoma and hypertrophic pulmonary osteoarthropathy. *Thorax*, **20**, 537.

an undifferentiated tumour with mediastinal glandular metastases) five years after pneumonectomy; and two (both with squamous tumours without mediastinal glandular metastases) six and seven years, respectively, after pneumonectomy. None survived after lobectomy. There were four operative deaths—two from pulmonary embolism after lobectomy; one (the only woman) from contralateral pulmonary infection after pneumonectomy; and one with congestive cardiac failure after lobectomy. Fourteen patients had died with metastases within a year of pulmonary resection—six more within two years, and the last four in this group within three years of pulmonary resection. In two patients in whom pulmonary resection was undertaken death was not related to metastases; one man died with purulent bronchitis six months after pneumonectomy, and the second died from coronary thrombosis six years after pneumonectomy; in neither instance were metastases found at necropsy.

The patient whose tumour was found to be inoperable died seven months after thoracotomy; of those irradiated two died during treatment and the remainder all within a year of treatment, six within six months.

Metastases in the 24 patients in whom these were the cause of death were clinically extra-thoracic in 20; in none of these patients did the clinical features of hypertrophic pulmonary osteoarthropathy recur. In four patients intrathoracic metastases were radiographically evident, and in two of these, with multiple peripheral pulmonary opacities later shown histologically to be caused by metastases, the clinical features of hypertrophic pulmonary osteoarthropathy recurred in the interval between one out-patient review, when the radiographic appearances of the remaining lung were normal, and the next, when metastases were demonstrated radiographically. The interval between radiographs in one patient was six months and in the other nine months. In both, symptoms prompted an earlier return for review than had been arranged, and both had tolerated joint pain and swelling for five or six weeks before seeking advice.

None of the large number of patients whose surgically managed primary tumour was not originally associated with hypertrophic pulmonary osteoarthropathy and who later developed intra-thoracic recurrence, either ipsilateral or contralateral, pleural or pulmonary, is known to have developed hypertrophic pulmonary osteoarthropathy in relation to tumour recurrence or metastasis.

Of 49 patients with hypertrophic pulmonary osteoarthropathy, therefore, a resection was undertaken in 34, exploration alone in one, and no operative procedure was undertaken in 14. Of those not managed by resection, all had died within a year of investigation. Of those managed by resection, there were four operative deaths; four were alive five years after pneumonectomy, but one of these has since died from coronary thrombosis; one is alive two years after pneumonectomy; 24 have died from metastases, all within three years of resection; the last of the group has died from infection, without metastasis, within a year of resection.

It is artificial to inflate small numbers to a percentage, but for ease of comparison, it may be said that, in the group of patients with a pulmonary tumour and hypertrophic pulmonary osteoarthropathy the tumour was operable in 69 per cent, whereas in only 36·6 per cent of those with pulmonary carcinoma without hypertrophic pulmonary osteoarthropathy was the tumour operable. In those with hypertrophic pulmonary osteoarthropathy the tumour was peripheral, again, in 69 per cent, and this is also a significantly higher proportion of peripheral tumours than in the series as a whole. The incidence of long survival was less than 8 per cent overall, 12 per cent in those submitted to resection and 13 per cent of those who survived resection.

SUMMARY

1. 4,000 patients with bronchial carcinoma, managed over a period of 15 years, are reviewed; 10 per cent (403 patients) were women.
2. Most patients were in the sixth and seventh decades. The incidence of the disease amongst those over 70 years is rising, and amongst those under 50 may be falling.
3. 15 per cent of patients were coal miners, an occupational incidence which may be disproportionately high; the survey was made in a region where coal mining is a common occupation.
4. 73 per cent of patients were known to smoke cigarettes; 4 per cent claimed never to have smoked; 15 per cent of women claimed never to have smoked; in a third of those who did not smoke the tumour was squamous.
5. Presentation in most cases was with respiratory symptoms or with an abnormal routine chest radiograph, symptoms being absent, or with clinical evidence of metastasis; 57 per cent had haemoptysis; daily haemoptysis and recurring febrile respiratory illness without complete recovery between episodes were the two most typical histories.
6. Investigation was on conventional lines in all well enough to withstand it. In three patients the chest radiograph was normal.
7. In 7 per cent of patients there was a related cardiovascular abnormality, sufficiently gross in one-tenth of these to preclude surgical management. Operative mortality was quadrupled in those with systemic hypertension with ECG changes, or with a history of angina of effort or previous coronary thrombosis.
8. 44·6 per cent of patients were regarded, after investigation, as suitable for exploratory thoracotomy with a view to management of pulmonary carcinoma by pulmonary resection. Pulmonary resection was completed in 36·6 per cent and abandoned because it was technically impossible or pointless in 8 per cent.
9. 45·9 per cent of patients had clinical, radiographic, fluoroscopic, bronchoscopic or thoracoscopic evidence of metastasis when first they were seen, or died during investigation.
10. 9·5 per cent of patients were unsuitable for surgical management for reasons other than metastatic.
11. A histological diagnosis was never established in 232 patients (5·7 per cent); in these the diagnosis of bronchial carcinoma, unsuitable for surgical management was beyond reasonable doubt.
12. The tumour was squamous in 1,946 patients (48·9 per cent); undifferentiated, including oat-cell, in 1,593 patients (39·8 per cent); adenocarcinoma in 212 (5·5 per cent); and an alveolar-cell carcinoma in 17 patients (0·4 per cent).
13. For the purpose of calculation, mixed tumours are included proportionately with one of the more definitive categories.

14. Amongst those tumours managed surgically, 62 per cent were squamous and 27 per cent undifferentiated.
15. Amongst those tumours found unsuitable for resection at exploratory thoracotomy, 51 per cent were squamous and 44 per cent undifferentiated.
16. Amongst those tumours found unsuitable for management by exploratory thoracotomy, 38 per cent were squamous and 48 per cent undifferentiated.
17. The operative mortality of exploration without resection was 6 per cent. Nearly three-quarters of those found by exploration to have irresectable tumours had died within a year of operation.
18. Pneumonectomy was undertaken in 24 per cent of patients. In 41 per cent of these hilar glands were invaded. The operative mortality of pneumonectomy was 12 per cent; the operative mortality rate increased significantly with age, and was 20 per cent in those 65 years or older. The operative mortality for right pneumonectomy was nearly twice that of left pneumonectomy.
19. The three common causes of death in the post-operative period after pneumonectomy were pulmonary infection, coronary thrombosis and pulmonary embolism—together accounting for three-quarters of the deaths in this group.
20. Survival rate in the first three years after pneumonectomy was significantly higher in those for whom resection was undertaken for squamous carcinoma than in those for whom resection was undertaken for undifferentiated carcinoma.
21. One in every three patients who died from metastases in the first two years after pneumonectomy died with cerebral metastases.
22. Of all patients submitted to pneumonectomy for bronchial carcinoma 24 per cent are alive, all more than two years after operation; 20 per cent of those submitted to pneumonectomy more than five years ago are alive.
23. Lobectomy was undertaken in 12 per cent of patients, in 65 per cent of these for squamous tumours. The operative mortality for lobectomy was 7 per cent overall, 14 per cent in those 65 years and older, and 22 per cent in those 70 years and older. Right upper lobectomy was the operation with the highest mortality rate in this group; " sleeve " resection was uncomplicated in 61 patients.
24. Of all patients submitted to lobectomy for bronchial carcinoma 47 per cent are alive, all more than two years after operation; 38 per cent of those submitted to lobectomy more than five years ago are alive and well.
25. Segmental resection was undertaken for bronchial carcinoma in 17 patients; five of these are long survivors.
26. Those patients who presented without symptoms, and with an abnormal chest radiograph made for an unrelated purpose were more often suitable for surgical management of bronchial carcinoma than were those who presented because of symptoms—but not all were suitable.
27. The number of patients with peripheral tumours was substantially higher and the number of patients with undifferentiated tumours substantially lower

amongst the group of patients who presented without symptoms and with an abnormality demonstrated on a routine chest radiograph made for unrelated purpose. Furthermore, only 26 per cent of this group were unsuitable for or declined thoracotomy as a form of management; operative mortality (5 per cent), and the rate of irresectability (5 per cent) were also lower, and the long survival rate (40 per cent) for all resections was higher, than in the series as a whole.

28. There was an 18 per cent error in the interpretation of peripheral pulmonary shadows the standard investigation of which was uninformative and subsequent management of which was by exploratory thoracotomy and diagnostic pulmonary resection. Diagnostic pulmonary resection was either unnecessary or of an unnecessary magnitude in 6·5 per cent of patients with peripheral pulmonary lesions of the variety defined. Some of these resections might have been avoided if skilled interpretation of frozen sections had constantly been available.

29. About one in four clinically palpable cervical glands resected for the purpose of biopsy in patients with bronchial carcinoma were shown not to be the site of metastasis.

30. In 10·6 per cent of the series a cervical node on the same side as the primary pulmonary tumour was the site of metastasis; in 1·9 per cent of the series bilateral cervical glandular metastases were demonstrated and in another 1·9 per cent only contralateral cervical glandular metastases were found.

31. In 45 per cent of patients with an ipsilateral cervical glandular metastasis this was the only evidence on standard clinical and special investigation of metastasis. A cervical lymph-glandular metastasis was the commonest clinical evidence of dissemination of bronchial carcinoma.

32. Cervical glandular metastasis from a left pulmonary primary, not only in the lower lobe, to the right side of the neck was only a little more common than was metastasis from a right pulmonary carcinoma to left cervical glands.

33. Bilateral cervical glandular metastases were only occasionally the only evidence of spread of bronchial carcinoma, and most patients with this evidence of dissemination died within six months of investigation, many within six weeks.

34. Axillary lymph-glandular metastases from bronchial carcinoma without chest wall invasion were the only clinical evidence of metastasis in 12 patients, in two of whom primary tumour and axillary gland were on opposite sides.

35. A radiographic opacity in the vicinity of the azygos vein and inseparable from the mediastinum in a patient with right or left bronchial carcinoma is good evidence of lymph-glandular metastasis and of unsuitability for surgical management.

36. Lymphangitis carcinomatosa in 24 patients was the only evidence of dissemination of tumour in seven of these, and was unilateral on the side of the tumour in six patients.

37. Presentation in 3·3 per cent of patients was with cerebral metastases. Hemiplegia, epilepsy and personality change were the three most common forms of presentation; speech defect, cerebellar symptoms and headache were other common reasons for presentation.

38. One of seven patients managed by craniotomy with excision of a cerebral metastasis and then resection of the primary pulmonary tumour is alive five years after completion of surgical management.

39. Where suspicion, however slight, is raised regarding the presence of cerebral metastases, the presence of which is unconfirmed by detailed investigation, the passage of time, often brief, usually confirms this suspicion.

40. In 2 per cent of patients osseous metastases were the only evidence of tumour spread at the time of first investigation; three in every four of these patients presented with the complaint of bone pain and without new respiratory symptoms.

41. The commonest sites of osseous metastases were the ribs and vertebrae.

42. Hepatic metastases were the only evidence of spread at the time of first investigation in 1·6 per cent of patients.

43. In 1 per cent of patients there were pulmono-pulmonary metastases at the time of first investigation as the only evidence of dissemination of tumour.

44. Pulmono-pulmonary metastasis from squamous carcinoma was relatively more common than from tumours of other histological type.

45. Unilateral pulmono-pulmonary metastases were more often contralateral than ipsilateral.

46. The diagnosis of pulmono-pulmonary metastases in patients with other causes for multiple pulmonary opacities, such as pneumoconiosis was, in some, achieved only after pulmonary biopsy.

47. At the time of first presentation 4·6 per cent of patients had the clinical features of obstruction of the superior vena cava. More (14 per cent) of these patients were women, average age was younger, and the incidence of undifferentiated tumours higher than in the series as a whole.

48. Obstruction of the superior vena cava and cervical lymph-glandular metastases, bilateral disproportionately often, were commonly associated.

49. Right vocal cord palsy was rare, and was found usually in association with obstruction of the superior vena cava and a right upper pulmonary carcinoma.

50. It was usually possible quickly to relieve the symptoms and signs of obstruction of the superior vena cava by irradiation; recurrence of caval obstruction was common and usually a herald of death.

51. Obstruction of the superior vena cava was nearly always associated with a right pulmonary carcinoma, usually in the right upper lobe.

52. Displacement of the barium-filled oesophagus accepted as evidence of mediastinal glandular metastasis was the only contra-indication to surgical management in 3·4 per cent of patients with bronchial carcinoma.

53. Dysphagia the consequence of malignant disease, where this is not a primary tumour in the proximal part of the alimentary tract, is usually from oesopha-

139

geal compression by mediastinal glands in which there are metastases from bronchial carcinoma.

54. Phrenic paresis was the only evidence of extension of tumour beyond the lung in 1·6 per cent of patients.

55. Interruption of the left recurrent laryngeal nerve was the only evidence of tumour spread in 3·3 per cent of patients.

56. The pulmonary opacity in patients with left recurrent laryngeal nerve palsy was left-sided in all but nine and in the left upper lobe or at the left hilum in two-thirds of those with left-sided tumours. Histological confirmation of the diagnosis of bronchial carcinoma was achieved in only one-third of the patients with left cord palsy at the time of their first investigation. Where the histology of the tumour was sooner or later established, squamous tumours predominated. Survival time from the onset of hoarseness of voice was often surprisingly long.

57. In 1 per cent of patients there were cutaneous or subcutaneous metastases as the only evidence of tumour dissemination at the time of first investigation.

58. Proximal extension of tumour, seen at bronchoscopy and established by biopsy precluded surgical management in 4·5 per cent of patients. Adenocarcinoma rarely extended in this way. A disproportionately large number of tumours which extended proximally were right-sided.

59. Invasion of the chest wall was recognised clinically and/or radiographically in 3·3 per cent of patients. In a third of these resection was undertaken because chest wall invasion was lateral; in another third the tumour was apical and associated with the features of Pancoast's syndrome; in the last third invasion was medial, either anteriorly or posteriorly.

60. Pleural effusion was routinely investigated by thoracoscopy, a technique which demonstrated the presence of pleural metastases as the only evidence of extrapulmonary extension of bronchial carcinoma in 2·1 per cent of patients.

61. Half the number of patients with pleural metastases had peripheral tumours, and a quarter were women. Adenocarcinoma metastasised to the pleura disproportionately often.

62. Most patients with pleural metastases had died within six months of the diagnosis having been made, as opposed to the not uncommon long survival in patients with primary pleural tumours.

63. Pleural effusion, even if sanguinous, in association with bronchial carcinoma is not synonymous with pleural metastasis. It is an indication for investigation, not a reason for despair.

64. Empyema thoracis co-existed with bronchial carcinoma or occurred as a complication of an operation for bronchial carcinoma in 1·4 per cent of patients. Empyema complicated pneumonectomy in 2·3 per cent of patients.

65. Relatively conservative management of empyema which complicated pneumonectomy—that is, management without thoracoplasty—was often successful.

66. Survival of patients in whom a resection for bronchial carcinoma had been complicated by empyema was sometimes surprisingly long; and of some continues.
67. Hypertrophic pulmonary osteoarthropathy was a concomitant of bronchial carcinoma in 1·2 per cent of patients. In this group of patients adenocarcinoma was represented disproportionately often.
68. The incidence of peripheral tumours and the rate of resectability among patients who presented with hypertrophic pulmonary osteoarthropathy was disproportionately high, and the incidence of long survival disproportionately low.
69. Resection of the pulmonary lesion, or irradiation relieved joint pain. The appearance of intra-thoracic recurrence or metastasis in the late postoperative period was, in two patients who presented with hypertrophic pulmonary osteoarthropathy, associated with the return of symptoms and signs of this concomitant of bronchial carcinoma. Hypertrophic pulmonary osteoarthropathy with recurrent tumour was never observed in patients who had not initially presented with hypertrophic pulmonary osteoarthropathy.
70. Diminished respiratory reserve was the only reason for not managing bronchial carcinoma surgically in 2·9 per cent of patients. More than three-quarters of the patients in this group were older than 59 years, whereas in the series as a whole fewer than half were older than 59 years.
71. In elderly patients with poor respiratory reserve and small peripheral tumours, death with, rather than from, bronchial carcinoma was thought often to have occurred.
72. In 3·5 per cent of patients a non-metastatic contra-indication to surgical management other than diminution in respiratory reserve was found—extensive pulmonary tuberculosis, asthma, gross pneumoconiosis, bullous emphysema, myocardial disease, age or frailty.
73. The development of an arrhythmia in a patient known to have bronchial carcinoma is likely to be significant of cardiac invasion.
74. 2 per cent of patients declined treatment, some of these also declining detailed investigation. As far as could be judged, all these patients were suitable candidates for management of bronchial carcinoma by pulmonary resection.
75. In 1·9 per cent of patients investigation was cut short by death—in many of these by a terminal event not directly attributable to bronchial carcinoma; most had evidence at necropsy of widespread metastasis. Techniques used in the investigation of 4,000 patients with bronchial carcinoma resulted in the death of two patients—a mortality from investigation of 0·05 per cent.

Index

INDEX

Printed by The Central Press (Aberdeen) Ltd.